Arthritis

The Complete Handbook for Sufferers and Caregivers

Ethan D. Anderson

Xspurts.com

A New Zealand Designed Product

Other Versions Available

Why limit yourself to just one format?

This book is now available in physical, digital, and audiobook options.

Choose the way you love to read and dive into the story today. You won't regret it!

Digital ISBN: 9781776967957
Physical ISBN: 9781776967940
Audio ISBN:

To obtain a different format of this book at a discounted price, please get in touch with us at:

http://isbn.xspurts.com/

Contents

Have Questions / Comments?

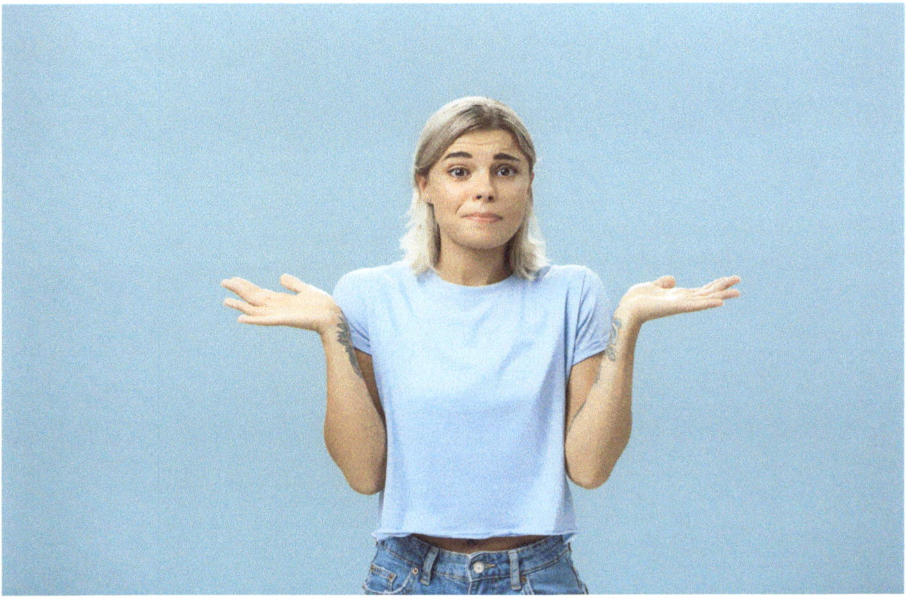

This book was designed to cover as much information as possible, but I know I have probably missed something, or some new amazing discovery has just come out.

If you notice something missing or have a question that I failed to answer, please get in touch and let me know. If I can, I will email you an answer and also update the book so others can also benefit from it.

Thanks For Being Awesome :)

Submit Your Questions / Comments At:

https://questions.xspurts.com

Get Free Stuff

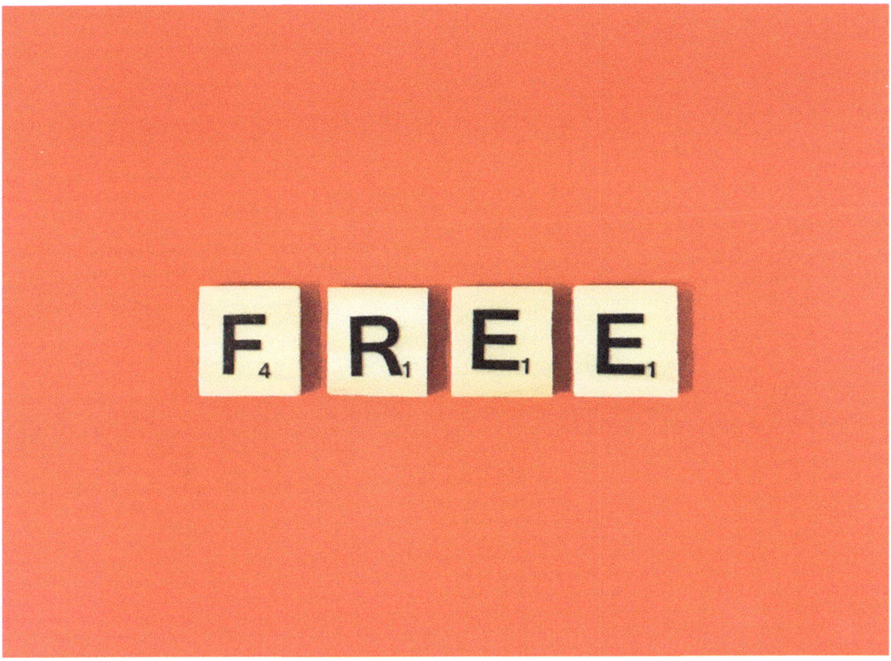

We love writing and have produced a huge number of books.

For being one of our amazing readers, we would love to offer you more books we have created, 100% free.

To claim this limited time special offer, simply go to the site below and enter your name and email address.

You will then receive loads (as we love our readers so much :) of our great books, content and audio direct to your email account, 100% free!

Get Loads of FREE Stuff at:

https://free.xspurts.com

Chapter One

Understanding Arthritis

Arthritis is a term used to describe joint inflammation and can refer to more than 100 different conditions that cause pain, stiffness, and swelling in the joints. It is a common problem that affects millions of people around the world, with the most common form being osteoarthritis.

Osteoarthritis is a degenerative joint disease that typically affects the elderly, although it can also occur in younger people who have suffered joint injuries or have a genetic predisposition to the condition. The condition is characterized by the gradual breakdown of cartilage, the connective tissue that cushions the joints, leading to pain, stiffness, and reduced mobility. While osteoarthritis is typically seen in weight-bearing joints such as the hips, knees, and spine, it can also affect the hands, fingers, and other joints.

Rheumatoid arthritis is another common type of arthritis, which is an autoimmune disorder that affects the joints. In this condition, the immune system mistakenly attacks the synovium, the lining of the joint capsule that produces the synovial fluid that lubricates the joints. This leads to inflammation, pain, and stiffness in the joints. Rheumatoid arthritis can also cause fatigue, fever, and weight loss, and it can lead to joint deformities over time.

Gout is another type of arthritis that occurs when there is a buildup of uric acid crystals in the joints, leading to inflammation and pain. This condition often affects the big toe, but it can also affect other joints in the body.

Other forms of arthritis include psoriatic arthritis, which affects people with psoriasis, an autoimmune skin condition, and ankylosing spondylitis, which primarily affects the spine and can lead to chronic pain and stiffness.

Arthritis is a complex condition with a variety of causes, including genetics, lifestyle factors, and environmental factors. While there is no cure for arthritis, there are many treatments available to manage the symptoms and improve quality of life for people with the condition.

Some common treatments for arthritis include medication, physical therapy, and lifestyle changes. Medications such as nonsteroidal anti-inflammatory drugs (NSAIDs), corticosteroids, and disease-modifying antirheumatic drugs (DMARDs) can help reduce inflammation and pain in the joints. Physical therapy can help improve mobility and strengthen the muscles around the affected joints, while lifestyle changes such as exercise, weight management, and a healthy diet can also help manage symptoms.

In some cases, surgery may be necessary to repair or replace damaged joints. Joint replacement surgery is a common procedure for people with severe osteoarthritis or other forms of arthritis that have not responded to other treatments.

Preventing arthritis is not always possible, but there are some steps that people can take to reduce their risk. Maintaining a healthy weight, staying physically active, and avoiding joint injuries can help prevent the development of osteoarthritis. Quitting smoking and reducing alcohol consumption can also help reduce the risk of developing certain types of arthritis.

The different types of arthritis

Arthritis is a broad term used to describe joint inflammation and can refer to more than 100 different conditions that cause pain, stiffness, and swelling in the joints. While there are many different types of arthritis, some of the most common include osteoarthritis, rheumatoid arthritis, gout, psoriatic arthritis, and ankylosing spondylitis.

Osteoarthritis is the most common form of arthritis, affecting millions of people around the world. It is a degenerative joint disease that typically occurs in older adults but can also affect younger people who have suffered joint injuries or have a genetic predisposition to the condition. Osteoarthritis is characterized by the gradual breakdown of cartilage, the connective tissue that cushions the joints, leading to pain, stiffness, and reduced mobility. While osteoarthritis is typically seen in weight-bearing joints such as the hips, knees, and spine, it can also affect the hands, fingers, and other joints.

Rheumatoid arthritis is another common type of arthritis, affecting about 1.3 million Americans. It is an autoimmune disorder in which the immune system mistakenly attacks the synovium, the lining of the joint capsule that produces the synovial fluid that lubricates the joints. This leads to inflammation, pain, and stiffness in the joints, and over time can cause joint damage and deformity. Rheumatoid arthritis can also cause fatigue, fever, and weight loss.

Gout is a type of arthritis that is caused by the buildup of uric acid crystals in the joints, leading to inflammation and pain. Gout often affects the big toe, but it can also affect other joints in the body. Gout is more common in men than women, and risk factors include obesity, high blood pressure, and kidney disease.

Psoriatic arthritis is a type of arthritis that affects some people with psoriasis, an autoimmune skin condition. Psoriatic arthritis can cause joint pain, stiffness, and swelling, and it can also cause nail changes and eye problems.

The severity of psoriatic arthritis can vary widely, from mild joint pain to severe joint damage and disability.

Ankylosing spondylitis is a type of arthritis that primarily affects the spine, but it can also affect other joints in the body. It is a chronic inflammatory disease that can lead to chronic pain and stiffness, and over time can cause the spine to fuse together. Ankylosing spondylitis is more common in men than women, and it usually starts in early adulthood.

Other less common types of arthritis include reactive arthritis, which can develop after an infection in the body; juvenile idiopathic arthritis, which affects children; and lupus, an autoimmune disorder that can cause joint pain and inflammation.

While each type of arthritis has its own unique characteristics, there are some common symptoms that people with arthritis may experience, including joint pain, stiffness, swelling, and reduced mobility. Many people with arthritis also experience fatigue, fever, and weight loss, and in some cases, arthritis can also affect other parts of the body, such as the eyes, skin, and internal organs.

Treatment for arthritis depends on the type and severity of the condition. For many people, medication is an important part of arthritis treatment, including nonsteroidal anti-inflammatory drugs (NSAIDs), corticosteroids, and disease-modifying antirheumatic drugs (DMARDs). Physical therapy can also be helpful for people with arthritis, as it can help improve mobility and strengthen the muscles around the affected joints. In some cases, surgery may be necessary to repair or replace damaged joints.

Preventing arthritis is not always possible, but there are some steps that people can take to reduce their risk. Maintaining a healthy weight, staying physically active, and avoiding joint injuries can

The role of inflammation

Inflammation is a natural process that occurs in the body as a response to injury, infection, or other forms of damage. While inflammation is a crucial part of the body's healing process, chronic inflammation can be harmful and can contribute to the development of many chronic diseases, including arthritis.

Arthritis is a broad term used to describe joint inflammation and can refer to more than 100 different conditions that cause pain, stiffness, and swelling in the joints. While there are many different types of arthritis, one common factor among many of them is inflammation.

Inflammation in the joints can cause pain, stiffness, and swelling, and over time, can lead to joint damage and deformity. Inflammation in the joints is caused by the immune system, which sends immune cells and other substances to the affected area to fight off infection or injury.

In some cases, however, the immune system can become overactive and mistakenly attack healthy tissues in the body, leading to chronic inflammation. In autoimmune diseases such as rheumatoid arthritis, the immune system mistakenly attacks the synovium, the lining of the joint capsule that produces the synovial fluid that lubricates the joints. This leads to inflammation, pain, and stiffness in the joints, and over time, can cause joint damage and deformity.

In addition to autoimmune diseases, other factors that can contribute to chronic inflammation in the body include a poor diet, lack of exercise, stress, and exposure to environmental toxins. These factors can cause the body to produce excess amounts of pro-inflammatory molecules, such as cytokines, which can contribute to inflammation in the joints and other parts of the body.

While inflammation is a natural part of the body's healing process, chronic inflammation can be harmful and can contribute to the development of many chronic diseases, including arthritis. In order to manage inflammation and reduce the risk of developing arthritis or other chronic diseases, there are several steps that people can take.

One of the most important steps is to maintain a healthy diet that is rich in anti-inflammatory foods such as fruits, vegetables, whole grains, and healthy fats. These foods contain nutrients and compounds that can help reduce inflammation in the body and promote overall health.

Regular exercise is also important for reducing inflammation and promoting joint health. Exercise helps to improve circulation, reduce stress, and strengthen the muscles around the joints, which can help support the joints and reduce the risk of injury.

Reducing stress and getting enough sleep are also important for managing inflammation and promoting overall health. Chronic stress can contribute to inflammation in the body, while getting enough sleep is important for regulating the immune system and promoting healing.

In addition to these lifestyle factors, there are also several natural remedies that can help reduce inflammation in the body. Some of these include turmeric, ginger, omega-3 fatty acids, and probiotics, all of which have been shown to have anti-inflammatory properties.

While inflammation is a natural process in the body, chronic inflammation can be harmful and can contribute to the development of many chronic diseases, including arthritis. By taking steps to reduce inflammation through a healthy diet, regular exercise, stress management, and natural remedies, people can help reduce their risk of developing arthritis and other chronic diseases, and promote overall health and well-being.

Symptoms and diagnosis

Arthritis is a broad term used to describe joint inflammation and can refer to more than 100 different conditions that cause pain, stiffness, and swelling in the joints. While each type of arthritis has its own unique characteristics, there are some common symptoms that people with arthritis may experience, as well as methods for diagnosis.

Symptoms of Arthritis:

Joint pain and stiffness are the most common symptoms of arthritis. Pain can be described as a dull ache or sharp sensation, and may be present both at rest and during movement. Stiffness can make it difficult to move the affected joint, particularly after periods of inactivity such as sleeping or sitting for long periods of time.

Swelling and redness may also be present in the affected joint or joints. Swelling is caused by an accumulation of fluid in the joint, and can cause a visible bulge or lump. Redness is caused by increased blood flow to the affected area.

Other symptoms of arthritis may include:

Reduced range of motion in the affected joint

Weakness or instability in the joint

Fatigue or general feeling of malaise

Fever or chills (particularly in cases of systemic arthritis)

Diagnosis of Arthritis:

Diagnosis of arthritis typically begins with a physical exam and medical history. During the physical exam, the doctor will evaluate the affected joint or joints, looking for signs of swelling, redness, and range of motion. The doctor may also perform specific tests to assess joint function and stability.

Blood tests may also be ordered to help diagnose arthritis. Tests can help identify markers of inflammation in the body, such as C-reactive protein (CRP) and erythrocyte sedimentation rate (ESR), which can be elevated in cases of arthritis.

Imaging tests such as X-rays, computed tomography (CT) scans, and magnetic resonance imaging (MRI) may also be used to help diagnose arthritis. Imaging tests can help identify joint damage or abnormalities, such as cartilage loss or bone spurs, which can be indicative of arthritis.

In some cases, joint fluid analysis may be performed to help diagnose arthritis. During this procedure, a needle is inserted into the affected joint, and a small amount of fluid is withdrawn and sent to a laboratory for analysis. This test can help identify the presence of inflammatory cells, which can indicate arthritis.

Diagnosis of arthritis can be challenging, as many of the symptoms are nonspecific and can be caused by a variety of other conditions. It is important for people with joint pain and stiffness to see a doctor if they are experiencing persistent symptoms, as early diagnosis and treatment can help prevent further joint damage and improve quality of life.

Chapter Two

Risk Factors and Causes

Arthritis is a broad term used to describe joint inflammation and can refer to more than 100 different conditions that cause pain, stiffness, and swelling in the joints. While the exact causes of arthritis are not well understood, there are several risk factors and underlying causes that have been identified.

Risk Factors:

1. Age: As people age, the risk of developing arthritis increases. Osteoarthritis, the most common form of arthritis, is more common in older adults, although it can also occur in younger people who have suffered joint injuries or have a genetic predisposition to the condition.

2. Gender: Some types of arthritis are more common in women than men, including rheumatoid arthritis and lupus. Gout, on the other hand, is more common in men than women.

3. Genetics: Some types of arthritis, such as rheumatoid arthritis, have a genetic component. People with a family history of arthritis are more likely to develop the condition themselves.

4. Obesity: Excess weight puts extra stress on the joints, particularly weight-bearing joints such as the hips, knees, and spine. This can increase the risk of developing osteoarthritis.

5. Joint injuries: Injuries to the joints, such as those caused by sports or accidents, can increase the risk of developing arthritis later in life.

6. Occupation: Jobs that require repetitive motions or heavy lifting can increase the risk of developing arthritis, particularly in the joints that are most frequently used.

Underlying Causes:

7. Inflammation: Chronic inflammation in the body can contribute to the development of arthritis. In autoimmune diseases such as rheumatoid arthritis, the immune system mistakenly attacks the synovium, the lining of the joint capsule that produces the synovial fluid that lubricates the joints. This leads to inflammation, pain, and stiffness in the joints, and over time, can cause joint damage and deformity.

8. Cartilage breakdown: In osteoarthritis, the most common form of arthritis, the gradual breakdown of cartilage in the joints leads to pain, stiffness, and reduced mobility.

9. Uric acid buildup: In gout, the buildup of uric acid crystals in the joints can cause inflammation and pain.

10. Infection: Some types of arthritis, such as reactive arthritis, can develop as a result of an infection in the body.

11. Environmental factors: Exposure to certain environmental factors, such as toxins and pollutants, can contribute to the development of arthritis.

While the exact causes of arthritis are not well understood, there are several risk factors and underlying causes that have been identified. By understanding these factors, people can take steps to reduce their risk of developing arthritis and manage their symptoms if they do develop the condition. Maintaining a healthy weight, staying physically active, avoiding joint injuries, and seeking early diagnosis and treatment can all help reduce the impact of arthritis on quality of life.

Genetic predisposition

Arthritis is a broad term used to describe joint inflammation and can refer to more than 100 different conditions that cause pain, stiffness, and swelling in the joints. While there are many different risk factors and underlying causes of arthritis, genetic predisposition is one factor that has been shown to play a significant role in the development of certain types of arthritis.

Genetic predisposition refers to an increased likelihood of developing a particular condition based on inherited genetic traits. In the case of arthritis, several genes have been identified that are associated with an increased risk of developing the condition.

One of the most well-known genetic risk factors for arthritis is the HLA gene. The HLA gene codes for proteins that play a role in the immune system, and certain variations of this gene have been associated with an increased risk of developing rheumatoid arthritis.

Other genes that have been associated with an increased risk of developing arthritis include:

1. STAT4: A gene that has been associated with an increased risk of developing rheumatoid arthritis and lupus

2. TRAF1/C5: A gene that has been associated with an increased risk of developing rheumatoid arthritis

3. IL-1: A gene that has been associated with an increased risk of developing osteoarthritis

While genetic predisposition is an important risk factor for arthritis, it is not the only factor. Environmental factors, such as diet, physical activity, and exposure to toxins and pollutants, can also play a role in the development of arthritis.

In some cases, genetic testing may be used to help diagnose and manage arthritis. Genetic testing can help identify specific genetic mutations or variations that are associated with an increased risk of developing arthritis. This information can be used to develop personalized treatment plans and to monitor the progression of the condition over time.

While there is no cure for arthritis, early diagnosis and treatment can help manage symptoms and prevent further joint damage. For people with a genetic predisposition to arthritis, early intervention may be particularly important. By understanding their risk and taking steps to manage their symptoms, people with a genetic predisposition to arthritis can help reduce the impact of the condition on their quality of life.

Environmental factors

Arthritis is a broad term used to describe joint inflammation and can refer to more than 100 different conditions that cause pain, stiffness, and swelling in the joints. While genetic predisposition is one risk factor for the development of arthritis, environmental factors also play an important role in the development of the condition.

Environmental factors refer to external factors that can impact health and can include a variety of different factors, such as diet, physical activity, exposure to toxins and pollutants, and stress. Several environmental factors have been identified that can contribute to the development of arthritis.

Diet:

Diet can play a significant role in the development and management of arthritis. Consuming a diet that is high in processed foods, saturated fats, and refined carbohydrates can contribute to chronic inflammation in the body, which can increase the risk of developing arthritis.

On the other hand, consuming a diet that is rich in anti-inflammatory foods, such as fruits, vegetables, whole grains, and healthy fats, can help reduce inflammation in the body and promote overall health.

Physical activity:

Regular physical activity is important for maintaining joint health and reducing the risk of developing arthritis. Exercise helps to improve joint flexibility and strength, and can help maintain a healthy weight, which can reduce the stress on joints.

However, certain types of exercise, such as high-impact activities or repetitive motions, can increase the risk of joint injury and may contribute to the development of arthritis in some cases.

Exposure to toxins and pollutants:

Exposure to certain toxins and pollutants, such as cigarette smoke, can contribute to the development of arthritis. Smoking has been shown to increase the risk of developing rheumatoid arthritis, and exposure to other toxins, such as heavy metals, has also been linked to an increased risk of developing the condition.

Stress:

Chronic stress can contribute to inflammation in the body, which can increase the risk of developing arthritis. Stress management techniques, such as mindfulness meditation and yoga, can help reduce stress and promote overall health.

In addition to these environmental factors, other factors that can contribute to the development of arthritis include joint injuries, infections, and certain medications.

By taking steps to reduce exposure to environmental factors that can contribute to the development of arthritis, people can help reduce their risk of developing the condition. Eating a healthy diet, staying physically active, avoiding exposure to toxins and pollutants, and practicing stress management techniques are all important for reducing the risk of arthritis and promoting overall health.

Lifestyle factors

Arthritis is a broad term used to describe joint inflammation and can refer to more than 100 different conditions that cause pain, stiffness, and swelling in the joints. While genetics and environmental factors can contribute to the development of arthritis, lifestyle factors such as diet, physical activity, and stress management can also play an important role in the management and prevention of the condition.

Diet:

Maintaining a healthy diet is important for managing arthritis symptoms and reducing inflammation in the body. A diet rich in fruits, vegetables, whole grains, and lean protein sources can provide the nutrients needed to maintain joint health and reduce inflammation.

In addition, certain foods have been shown to have anti-inflammatory properties, including fatty fish such as salmon and mackerel, nuts such as almonds and walnuts, and spices such as turmeric and ginger.

On the other hand, consuming a diet high in processed foods, refined carbohydrates, and saturated fats can contribute to chronic inflammation in the body and increase the risk of developing arthritis.

Physical activity:

Regular physical activity is important for maintaining joint health and reducing the risk of developing arthritis. Exercise can help improve joint flexibility and strength, as well as maintain a healthy weight, which can reduce the stress on joints.

It is important to choose activities that are appropriate for one's physical abilities and to gradually increase the intensity and duration of exercise over time. High-impact activities, such as running and jumping, may not be appropriate for everyone and can increase the risk of joint injury.

Stress management:

Stress can contribute to inflammation in the body, which can increase the risk of developing arthritis and exacerbate existing symptoms. Stress management techniques, such as mindfulness meditation and yoga, can help reduce stress and promote overall health.

Getting enough rest and prioritizing self-care can also help reduce stress and promote overall well-being.

Smoking:

Smoking has been shown to increase the risk of developing rheumatoid arthritis and can exacerbate symptoms in people who already have arthritis.

Quitting smoking can improve overall health and reduce the risk of developing arthritis or experiencing flare-ups of existing symptoms.

Alcohol consumption:

Excessive alcohol consumption can contribute to inflammation in the body and may exacerbate symptoms in people with arthritis. Limiting alcohol consumption can help reduce inflammation and improve overall health.

Chapter Three

Living with Arthritis

Arthritis is a chronic condition that can have a significant impact on daily life. While there is no cure for arthritis, there are many strategies that can help people manage their symptoms and maintain their quality of life.

Managing Pain:

Pain is one of the most common symptoms of arthritis and can be one of the most challenging to manage. There are several strategies that can help reduce pain and discomfort, including:

1. Heat and cold therapy: Applying heat or cold to the affected joint can help reduce pain and stiffness. Heat can help relax muscles and increase blood flow, while cold can help reduce inflammation and numb pain.

2. Exercise: Regular exercise can help improve joint flexibility and reduce pain. Low-impact activities such as swimming, walking, and cycling are often recommended for people with arthritis.

3. Medication: Over-the-counter pain relievers such as acetaminophen and nonsteroidal anti-inflammatory drugs (NSAIDs) can help reduce pain and inflammation. In some cases, prescription medications such as corticosteroids or biologic drugs may be necessary.

4. Massage: Massage can help reduce pain and stiffness in the joints and promote overall relaxation.

Managing Fatigue:

Fatigue is another common symptom of arthritis and can be caused by a variety of factors, including pain, inflammation, and medication side effects. There are several strategies that can help reduce fatigue and increase energy levels, including:

5. Rest: Getting enough rest and sleep is important for managing fatigue. It may be necessary to take short naps or breaks throughout the day to manage fatigue.

6. Exercise: Regular exercise can help improve energy levels and reduce fatigue. Low-impact activities such as walking or swimming may be particularly helpful.

7. Stress management: Managing stress can help reduce fatigue and promote relaxation. Techniques such as mindfulness meditation and deep breathing can be helpful.

8. Pace activities: It may be necessary to pace activities throughout the day to avoid overexertion and fatigue. Breaking tasks into smaller, manageable pieces and taking breaks as needed can help manage fatigue.

Managing Joint Stiffness:

Joint stiffness is a common symptom of arthritis and can be particularly challenging in the morning or after periods of inactivity. There are several strategies that can help reduce joint stiffness and improve mobility, including:

9. Gentle stretching: Gentle stretching can help improve joint flexibility and reduce stiffness. It is important to avoid overstretching or straining the joints.

10. Heat therapy: Applying heat to the affected joint can help relax muscles and improve joint flexibility.

11. Exercise: Regular exercise, particularly low-impact activities such as walking or swimming, can help improve joint mobility and reduce stiffness.

12. Medication: In some cases, medication such as NSAIDs or corticosteroids may be necessary to reduce joint stiffness and inflammation.

Making Lifestyle Changes:

In addition to managing specific symptoms of arthritis, making lifestyle changes can help improve overall health and reduce the impact of arthritis on quality of life. Some lifestyle changes that can be helpful include:

13. Maintaining a healthy weight: Excess weight can put stress on the joints and exacerbate arthritis symptoms. Maintaining a healthy weight can help reduce joint stress and improve overall health.

14. Eating a healthy diet: Eating a diet that is rich in anti-inflammatory foods, such as fruits, vegetables, whole grains, and healthy fats, can help reduce inflammation in the body and improve overall health.

15. Staying physically active: Regular exercise can help improve joint flexibility and reduce pain, stiffness, and fatigue.

16. Managing stress: Managing stress through techniques such as mindfulness meditation, deep breathing, or yoga can help reduce inflammation in the body and improve overall health.

Living with arthritis can be challenging, but there are many strategies that can help manage symptoms and improve quality of life. By managing pain, fatigue, and joint stiffness, making lifestyle changes, and seeking support from healthcare professionals, people

Coping with pain and stiffness

Arthritis is a chronic condition that can cause pain and stiffness in the joints, making it difficult to perform daily activities. Coping with pain and stiffness is an important aspect of managing arthritis and can help improve overall quality of life. Here are some strategies for coping with pain and stiffness associated with arthritis:

Heat and Cold Therapy:

Heat and cold therapy can be effective in reducing pain and stiffness in the joints. Applying a heating pad or warm towel to the affected joint can help increase blood flow and promote relaxation, while applying a cold compress can help reduce inflammation and numb pain. It is important to use heat or cold therapy as directed by a healthcare professional, as excessive use can cause tissue damage.

Exercise:

Regular exercise can help reduce pain and stiffness in the joints, as well as improve joint flexibility and overall physical function. Low-impact exercises such as swimming, walking, and cycling are often recommended for people with arthritis. It is important to consult with a healthcare professional before starting an exercise program, as they can help develop an appropriate plan that takes into account any joint damage or limitations.

Medications:

Over-the-counter pain relievers such as acetaminophen and nonsteroidal anti-inflammatory drugs (NSAIDs) can be effective in reducing pain and inflammation associated with arthritis. In some cases, prescription medications such as corticosteroids or biologic drugs may be necessary to manage severe symptoms.

Massage Therapy:

Massage therapy can help reduce pain and stiffness in the joints and promote relaxation. It is important to work with a licensed massage therapist who is familiar with arthritis and can tailor the massage to the individual's needs.

Stress Management:

Stress can contribute to inflammation in the body and exacerbate arthritis symptoms. Stress management techniques such as mindfulness meditation, deep breathing, or yoga can help reduce stress and promote relaxation.

Joint Protection:

Protecting the joints from further damage can help reduce pain and stiffness associated with arthritis. This can include using assistive devices such as braces or splints, modifying activities to avoid overuse of the joints, and maintaining good posture to reduce stress on the joints.

Diet:

Maintaining a healthy diet can help reduce inflammation in the body and improve overall health. Eating a diet that is rich in anti-inflammatory foods, such as fruits, vegetables, whole grains, and healthy fats, can be particularly helpful for people with arthritis.

Sleep:

Getting enough restful sleep is important for managing pain and stiffness associated with arthritis. It is important to establish a regular sleep routine, avoid caffeine and alcohol before bedtime, and create a comfortable sleeping environment.

Managing fatigue

Fatigue is a common symptom of arthritis and can have a significant impact on daily life. Managing fatigue is an important aspect of managing arthritis and can help improve overall quality of life. Here are some strategies for managing fatigue associated with arthritis:

Rest:

Getting enough rest and sleep is important for managing fatigue. It may be necessary to take short naps or breaks throughout the day to manage fatigue. Establishing a regular sleep routine can also help improve sleep quality.

Exercise:

Regular exercise can help improve energy levels and reduce fatigue. Low-impact activities such as walking, cycling, or swimming are often recommended for people with arthritis. It is important to consult with a healthcare professional before starting an exercise program, as they can help develop an appropriate plan that takes into account any joint damage or limitations.

Stress Management:

Stress can contribute to fatigue and exacerbate arthritis symptoms. Stress management techniques such as mindfulness meditation, deep breathing, or yoga can help reduce stress and promote relaxation.

Pacing Activities:

It may be necessary to pace activities throughout the day to avoid overexertion and fatigue. Breaking tasks into smaller, manageable pieces and taking breaks as needed can help manage fatigue.

Medications:

In some cases, medications such as antidepressants or stimulants may be necessary to manage severe fatigue associated with arthritis. It is important to work with a healthcare professional to determine the appropriate medication and dosage.

Diet:

Maintaining a healthy diet can help improve energy levels and reduce fatigue associated with arthritis. Eating a diet that is rich in fruits, vegetables, whole grains, and lean protein sources can provide the nutrients needed to maintain energy levels throughout the day.

Manage Pain:

Pain can contribute to fatigue and make it difficult to perform daily activities. Managing pain through medications, heat and cold therapy, and other strategies can help reduce fatigue and improve overall quality of life.

Support:

Living with arthritis can be challenging, and seeking support from friends, family, or a support group can help reduce stress and fatigue associated with the condition. It is important to talk openly about feelings and concerns and to seek help when needed.

Navigating relationships and emotional wellbeing

Arthritis can have a significant impact on emotional well-being and relationships. Coping with the physical symptoms of arthritis can be challenging, and managing the emotional and social impact of the condition is equally important. Here are some strategies for navigating relationships and emotional well-being when living with arthritis:

Communication:

Communication is key to maintaining healthy relationships when living with arthritis. It is important to talk openly with friends, family, and loved ones about the condition, how it affects daily life, and how they can offer support. This can help reduce stress and feelings of isolation.

Setting Boundaries:

Living with arthritis can require making adjustments to daily life and activities. Setting boundaries and saying "no" to activities or commitments that may exacerbate symptoms or cause stress can help manage the condition and improve emotional well-being.

Seeking Support:

Living with arthritis can be challenging, and seeking support from friends, family, or a support group can help reduce stress and feelings of isolation. It is important to talk openly about feelings and concerns and to seek help when needed.

Managing Stress:

Stress can exacerbate arthritis symptoms and impact emotional well-being. Managing stress through techniques such as mindfulness meditation, deep breathing, or yoga can help reduce stress and promote relaxation.

Maintaining Social Connections:

Arthritis can make it difficult to participate in social activities, but maintaining social connections is important for emotional well-being. It is important to find activities that are enjoyable and that can be done with friends and loved ones.

Counseling:

Living with a chronic condition like arthritis can be emotionally challenging. Seeking counseling or therapy can provide support and guidance for managing emotions and relationships.

Self-Care:

Self-care is important for emotional well-being when living with arthritis. Taking time for activities that promote relaxation and joy, such as reading, taking a bath, or spending time in nature, can help improve emotional well-being.

Advocating for Yourself:

Living with arthritis can require advocating for oneself in healthcare settings and in other areas of life. It is important to communicate with healthcare professionals about symptoms, concerns, and treatment options, and to take an active role in managing the condition.

Chapter Four

Medical Treatments

Arthritis is a chronic condition that affects millions of people worldwide. While there is no cure for arthritis, there are several medical treatments that can help manage symptoms and improve quality of life. Here are some of the most common medical treatments for arthritis:

Nonsteroidal Anti-Inflammatory Drugs (NSAIDs):

NSAIDs are a type of medication that help reduce pain and inflammation in the joints. Common NSAIDs include ibuprofen, naproxen, and aspirin. NSAIDs are available over-the-counter or by prescription and can be effective in managing mild to moderate arthritis symptoms.

Disease-Modifying Anti-Rheumatic Drugs (DMARDs):

DMARDs are a type of medication that work to slow down the progression of arthritis and reduce joint damage. DMARDs are often used in cases of rheumatoid arthritis and other autoimmune forms of arthritis. Common DMARDs include methotrexate, sulfasalazine, and hydroxychloroquine.

Biologic Drugs:

Biologic drugs are a newer class of medication that target specific molecules in the immune system to reduce inflammation and slow down the progression of arthritis. Biologic drugs are often used in cases of rheumatoid arthritis and other autoimmune forms of arthritis. Common biologic drugs include etanercept, adalimumab, and infliximab.

Corticosteroids:

Corticosteroids are a type of medication that help reduce inflammation and pain in the joints. Corticosteroids can be taken orally or injected directly into the affected joint. Corticosteroids are often used for short periods of time to manage acute arthritis symptoms.

Joint Injections:

Joint injections involve injecting medication directly into the affected joint to reduce inflammation and pain. Common medications used in joint injections include corticosteroids and hyaluronic acid. Joint injections are often used in cases of osteoarthritis.

Surgery:

In cases of severe arthritis, surgery may be necessary to replace or repair damaged joints. Common surgeries for arthritis include joint replacement surgery, joint fusion surgery, and joint repair surgery.

Physical Therapy:

Physical therapy can be an effective treatment for arthritis by improving joint flexibility and strength, reducing pain, and improving overall physical function. Physical therapy can include exercises, stretches, and other techniques to improve joint mobility and reduce stiffness.

Pain relievers

Arthritis is a chronic condition that can cause pain and stiffness in the joints, making it difficult to perform daily activities. Pain relievers are a common treatment for managing arthritis symptoms and improving quality of life. Here are some of the most common pain relievers used for arthritis:

Acetaminophen:

Acetaminophen is a pain reliever that is available over-the-counter and is used to manage mild to moderate arthritis pain. Acetaminophen works by reducing the brain's perception of pain, but it does not reduce inflammation in the joints.

Nonsteroidal Anti-Inflammatory Drugs (NSAIDs):

NSAIDs are a type of pain reliever that works by reducing pain and inflammation in the joints. NSAIDs are available over-the-counter or by prescription and can be effective in managing mild to moderate arthritis symptoms. Common NSAIDs include ibuprofen, naproxen, and aspirin.

Topical Pain Relievers:

Topical pain relievers are medications that are applied directly to the skin over the affected joint. Topical pain relievers can be effective in reducing pain and inflammation in the joints without causing side effects that are associated with oral medications. Common topical pain relievers include creams, gels, and patches that contain menthol, capsaicin, or salicylates.

Opioids:

Opioids are a type of pain reliever that are used to manage severe arthritis pain. Opioids are available by prescription and are often reserved for cases where other pain relievers have been ineffective. Opioids work by blocking pain signals in the brain, but they can be addictive and can cause side effects such as dizziness, nausea, and constipation.

Corticosteroids:

Corticosteroids are a type of medication that help reduce inflammation and pain in the joints. Corticosteroids can be taken orally or injected directly into the affected joint. Corticosteroids are often used for short periods of time to manage acute arthritis symptoms.

Hyaluronic Acid:

Hyaluronic acid is a type of medication that is injected directly into the affected joint to reduce pain and inflammation. Hyaluronic acid is a natural substance that is found in the joints and helps lubricate the joints. Hyaluronic acid injections are often used in cases of osteoarthritis.

Disease-Modifying Anti-Rheumatic Drugs (DMARDs):

DMARDs are a type of medication that work to slow down the progression of arthritis and reduce joint damage. DMARDs are often used in cases of rheumatoid arthritis and other autoimmune forms of arthritis. DMARDs can help reduce pain and inflammation in the joints over time.

Anti-inflammatory drugs

Arthritis is a chronic condition that causes inflammation in the joints, leading to pain and stiffness. Anti-inflammatory drugs are a common treatment for managing arthritis symptoms and reducing inflammation in the joints. Here are some of the most common anti-inflammatory drugs used for arthritis:

Nonsteroidal Anti-Inflammatory Drugs (NSAIDs):

NSAIDs are a type of medication that works by blocking the production of prostaglandins, which are chemicals in the body that cause inflammation and pain. NSAIDs can be effective in managing mild to moderate arthritis symptoms and reducing inflammation in the joints. Common NSAIDs include ibuprofen, naproxen, and aspirin.

Disease-Modifying Anti-Rheumatic Drugs (DMARDs):

DMARDs are a type of medication that work to slow down the progression of arthritis and reduce joint damage. DMARDs are often used in cases of rheumatoid arthritis and other autoimmune forms of arthritis. DMARDs can help reduce inflammation in the joints over time and prevent joint damage. Common DMARDs include methotrexate, sulfasalazine, and hydroxychloroquine.

Biologic Drugs:

Biologic drugs are a newer class of medication that target specific molecules in the immune system to reduce inflammation and slow down the progression of arthritis. Biologic drugs are often used in cases of rheumatoid arthritis and other autoimmune forms of arthritis. Common biologic drugs include etanercept, adalimumab, and infliximab.

Corticosteroids:

Corticosteroids are a type of medication that help reduce inflammation and pain in the joints. Corticosteroids can be taken orally or injected directly into the affected joint. Corticosteroids are often used for short periods of time to manage acute arthritis symptoms.

Colchicine:

Colchicine is a medication that is used to treat gout, which is a type of arthritis that is caused by the buildup of uric acid crystals in the joints. Colchicine works by reducing inflammation in the joints and preventing the formation of uric acid crystals. Colchicine can be effective in managing acute gout attacks.

Interleukin-1 Inhibitors:

Interleukin-1 inhibitors are a type of biologic drug that work by blocking the action of interleukin-1, which is a molecule that causes inflammation in the joints. Interleukin-1 inhibitors can be effective in managing symptoms of rheumatoid arthritis and other autoimmune forms of arthritis.

Janus Kinase (JAK) Inhibitors:

JAK inhibitors are a type of medication that work by blocking the action of Janus kinase enzymes, which are involved in the inflammation process in the body. JAK inhibitors can be effective in managing symptoms of rheumatoid arthritis and other autoimmune forms of arthritis. Common JAK inhibitors include tofacitinib and baricitinib.

Disease-modifying antirheumatic drugs (DMARDs)

Arthritis is a chronic condition that can cause pain, stiffness, and inflammation in the joints. Disease-modifying antirheumatic drugs (DMARDs) are a type of medication that work to slow down the progression of arthritis and reduce joint damage. Here are some important facts about DMARDs and their use in treating arthritis:

How do DMARDs work?

DMARDs work by suppressing the immune system, which is overactive in people with autoimmune forms of arthritis such as rheumatoid arthritis. DMARDs can help reduce inflammation in the joints and prevent joint damage over time. DMARDs are often used in combination with other medications such as nonsteroidal anti-inflammatory drugs (NSAIDs) to manage arthritis symptoms.

Types of DMARDs

There are several types of DMARDs available, including:

1. Methotrexate: Methotrexate is one of the most commonly used DMARDs for rheumatoid arthritis. Methotrexate works by inhibiting the growth of cells that contribute to inflammation in the joints.

2. Sulfasalazine: Sulfasalazine is another DMARD that is often used for rheumatoid arthritis. Sulfasalazine works by suppressing the immune system and reducing inflammation in the joints.

3. Hydroxychloroquine: Hydroxychloroquine is a DMARD that is used to treat rheumatoid arthritis and other autoimmune forms of arthritis. Hydroxychloroquine works by reducing inflammation in the joints and suppressing the immune system.

4. Leflunomide: Leflunomide is a DMARD that is used to treat rheumatoid arthritis. Leflunomide works by inhibiting the growth of cells that contribute to inflammation in the joints.

5. Biologic DMARDs: Biologic DMARDs are a newer class of medication that target specific molecules in the immune system to reduce inflammation and slow down the progression of arthritis. Biologic DMARDs are often used in cases of rheumatoid arthritis and other autoimmune forms of arthritis. Common biologic DMARDs include etanercept, adalimumab, and infliximab.

How are DMARDs administered?

DMARDs can be administered in several ways, including:

6. Oral tablets: Methotrexate, sulfasalazine, hydroxychloroquine, and leflunomide are all available in oral tablet form.

7. Injections: Biologic DMARDs are often administered via injection. The injections can be given by a healthcare professional or self-administered at home.

8. Infusions: Some biologic DMARDs are administered via infusion, which involves receiving the medication through an intravenous (IV) line.

Side effects of DMARDs

DMARDs can cause side effects, and it is important to work with a healthcare professional to monitor for these side effects. Common side effects of DMARDs include:

Nausea and vomiting

Diarrhea

Hair loss

Headache

Fatigue

Increased risk of infection

Liver damage

Monitoring and follow-up

It is important to have regular monitoring and follow-up with a healthcare professional when taking DMARDs. Blood tests and other diagnostic tests may be necessary to monitor for side effects and ensure that the medication is working effectively.

Chapter Five

Natural Remedies and Supplements

Arthritis is a chronic condition that can cause pain, stiffness, and inflammation in the joints. While there is no cure for arthritis, natural remedies and supplements can be effective in managing symptoms and improving overall quality of life. Here are some of the most common natural remedies and supplements used for arthritis:

Turmeric:

Turmeric is a spice that is commonly used in Indian and Middle Eastern cuisine. Turmeric contains a compound called curcumin, which has anti-inflammatory properties. Studies have shown that taking turmeric supplements can be effective in reducing joint pain and stiffness in people with osteoarthritis and rheumatoid arthritis.

Omega-3 Fatty Acids:

Omega-3 fatty acids are essential fatty acids that are found in fish such as salmon, tuna, and mackerel. Omega-3 fatty acids have anti-inflammatory properties and can be effective in reducing joint pain and stiffness in people with arthritis. Omega-3 supplements are also available and can be an effective natural remedy for managing arthritis symptoms.

Ginger:

Ginger is a root that has been used for thousands of years in traditional medicine. Ginger contains compounds called gingerols and shogaols, which have anti-inflammatory properties. Studies have shown that taking ginger supplements can be effective in reducing joint pain and stiffness in people with osteoarthritis and rheumatoid arthritis.

Glucosamine and Chondroitin:

Glucosamine and chondroitin are supplements that are often used together to manage arthritis symptoms. Glucosamine is a natural substance that is found in cartilage, while chondroitin is a natural substance that is found in the connective tissue of joints. Both supplements can be effective in reducing joint pain and stiffness in people with osteoarthritis.

Vitamin D:

Vitamin D is an essential nutrient that is important for bone health. Studies have shown that low levels of vitamin D can be associated with an increased risk of osteoarthritis and rheumatoid arthritis. Taking vitamin D supplements can be an effective way to manage arthritis symptoms and improve overall bone health.

Massage Therapy:

Massage therapy can be an effective natural remedy for managing arthritis symptoms. Massage therapy can help reduce pain and stiffness in the joints, improve range of motion, and improve overall quality of life for people with arthritis.

Exercise:

Regular exercise can be an effective way to manage arthritis symptoms and improve overall physical health. Exercise can help improve joint flexibility, reduce pain and stiffness in the joints, and improve overall muscle strength.

Herbal remedies

Arthritis is a chronic condition that can cause pain, stiffness, and inflammation in the joints. While there are several conventional treatments available for managing arthritis symptoms, some people turn to herbal remedies as an alternative or complementary approach. Here are some of the most commonly used herbal remedies for arthritis:

Boswellia:

Boswellia is an herb that is commonly used in traditional medicine. Boswellia contains compounds called boswellic acids, which have anti-inflammatory properties. Studies have shown that taking boswellia supplements can be effective in reducing joint pain and stiffness in people with osteoarthritis and rheumatoid arthritis.

Ginger:

Ginger is a root that has been used for thousands of years in traditional medicine. Ginger contains compounds called gingerols and shogaols, which have anti-inflammatory properties. Studies have shown that taking ginger supplements can be effective in reducing joint pain and stiffness in people with osteoarthritis and rheumatoid arthritis.

Turmeric:

Turmeric is a spice that is commonly used in Indian and Middle Eastern cuisine. Turmeric contains a compound called curcumin, which has anti-inflammatory properties. Studies have shown that taking turmeric supplements can be effective in reducing joint pain and stiffness in people with osteoarthritis and rheumatoid arthritis.

Cat's Claw:

Cat's claw is an herb that is native to South America. Cat's claw contains compounds called pentacyclic oxindole alkaloids, which have anti-inflammatory properties. Studies have shown that taking cat's claw supplements can be effective in reducing joint pain and stiffness in people with rheumatoid arthritis.

Green Tea:

Green tea is a type of tea that is commonly consumed in Asian countries. Green tea contains compounds called catechins, which have anti-inflammatory properties. Studies have shown that drinking green tea can be effective in reducing joint pain and stiffness in people with rheumatoid arthritis.

Devil's Claw:

Devil's claw is an herb that is native to southern Africa. Devil's claw contains compounds called harpagosides, which have anti-inflammatory properties. Studies have shown that taking devil's claw supplements can be effective in reducing joint pain and stiffness in people with osteoarthritis.

Willow Bark:

Willow bark is an herb that has been used for thousands of years in traditional medicine. Willow bark contains a compound called salicin, which is similar to aspirin and has anti-inflammatory properties. Studies have shown that taking willow bark supplements can be effective in reducing joint pain and stiffness in people with osteoarthritis and rheumatoid arthritis.

It is important to note that herbal remedies can have side effects and interact with other medications. It is important to work with a healthcare professional to determine the appropriate herbal remedies for managing arthritis symptoms and to monitor for any potential side effects or interactions.

Dietary supplements

Arthritis is a chronic condition that can cause pain, stiffness, and inflammation in the joints. While there are several conventional treatments available for managing arthritis symptoms, some people turn to dietary supplements as an alternative or complementary approach. Here are some of the most commonly used dietary supplements for arthritis:

Glucosamine and Chondroitin:

Glucosamine and chondroitin are supplements that are often used together to manage arthritis symptoms. Glucosamine is a natural substance that is found in cartilage, while chondroitin is a natural substance that is found in the connective tissue of joints. Both supplements can be effective in reducing joint pain and stiffness in people with osteoarthritis.

Omega-3 Fatty Acids:

Omega-3 fatty acids are essential fatty acids that are found in fish such as salmon, tuna, and mackerel. Omega-3 fatty acids have anti-inflammatory properties and can be effective in reducing joint pain and stiffness in people with arthritis. Omega-3 supplements are also available and can be an effective dietary supplement for managing arthritis symptoms.

Vitamin D:

Vitamin D is an essential nutrient that is important for bone health. Studies have shown that low levels of vitamin D can be associated with an increased risk of osteoarthritis and rheumatoid arthritis. Taking vitamin D supplements can be an effective way to manage arthritis symptoms and improve overall bone health.

Calcium:

Calcium is an essential nutrient that is important for bone health. Studies have shown that low levels of calcium can be associated with an increased risk of osteoarthritis and rheumatoid arthritis. Taking calcium supplements can be an effective way to manage arthritis symptoms and improve overall bone health.

SAMe:

SAMe, or S-adenosylmethionine, is a natural substance that is found in the body. SAMe supplements can be effective in reducing joint pain and stiffness in people with osteoarthritis. SAMe may also be effective in reducing the need for nonsteroidal anti-inflammatory drugs (NSAIDs) in people with osteoarthritis.

Probiotics:

Probiotics are beneficial bacteria that are found in the gut. Studies have shown that probiotics can be effective in reducing inflammation and improving overall immune function. Probiotic supplements can be an effective dietary supplement for managing arthritis symptoms.

Vitamin C:

Vitamin C is an essential nutrient that is important for immune function and collagen synthesis. Studies have shown that low levels of vitamin C can be associated with an increased risk of developing osteoarthritis. Taking vitamin C supplements can be an effective way to manage arthritis symptoms and improve overall immune function.

It is important to note that dietary supplements can have side effects and interact with other medications. It is important to work with a healthcare professional to determine the appropriate dietary supplements for managing arthritis symptoms and to monitor for any potential side effects or interactions.

Essential oils

Arthritis is a chronic condition that can cause pain, stiffness, and inflammation in the joints. While there are several conventional treatments available for managing arthritis symptoms, some people turn to essential oils as an alternative or complementary approach. Here are some of the most commonly used essential oils for arthritis:

Peppermint Oil:

Peppermint oil contains menthol, which has a cooling effect that can help reduce joint pain and stiffness. Peppermint oil can be applied topically or inhaled through aromatherapy to help manage arthritis symptoms.

Eucalyptus Oil:

Eucalyptus oil contains a compound called eucalyptol, which has anti-inflammatory and analgesic properties. Eucalyptus oil can be applied topically or inhaled through aromatherapy to help manage arthritis symptoms.

Ginger Oil:

Ginger oil contains compounds called gingerols and shogaols, which have anti-inflammatory properties. Ginger oil can be applied topically or inhaled through aromatherapy to help manage arthritis symptoms.

Frankincense Oil:

Frankincense oil contains a compound called boswellic acid, which has anti-inflammatory properties. Frankincense oil can be applied topically or inhaled through aromatherapy to help manage arthritis symptoms.

Lavender Oil:

Lavender oil has a calming effect and can help reduce stress and anxiety, which can exacerbate arthritis symptoms. Lavender oil can be applied topically or inhaled through aromatherapy to help manage arthritis symptoms.

Rosemary Oil:

Rosemary oil contains a compound called rosmarinic acid, which has anti-inflammatory and antioxidant properties. Rosemary oil can be applied topically or inhaled through aromatherapy to help manage arthritis symptoms.

Chamomile Oil:

Chamomile oil contains compounds called flavonoids, which have anti-inflammatory properties. Chamomile oil can be applied topically or inhaled through aromatherapy to help manage arthritis symptoms.

It is important to note that essential oils can have side effects and should be used with caution. Essential oils should be diluted before application and should not be ingested. It is also important to note that essential oils should not be used as a replacement for conventional medical treatment for arthritis.

Chapter Six

Nutrition and Diet

Arthritis is a chronic condition that can cause pain, stiffness, and inflammation in the joints. While there are several conventional treatments available for managing arthritis symptoms, nutrition and diet can also play an important role in managing the condition. Here are some nutrition and diet tips for managing arthritis:

Omega-3 Fatty Acids:

Omega-3 fatty acids are essential fatty acids that are found in fish such as salmon, tuna, and mackerel. Omega-3 fatty acids have anti-inflammatory properties and can be effective in reducing joint pain and stiffness in people with arthritis. Omega-3 supplements are also available and can be an effective dietary supplement for managing arthritis symptoms.

Vitamin D:

Vitamin D is an essential nutrient that is important for bone health. Studies have shown that low levels of vitamin D can be associated with an increased risk of osteoarthritis and rheumatoid arthritis. Vitamin D can be found in foods such as fatty fish, egg yolks, and fortified foods. It is also important to get adequate sunlight exposure to help the body produce vitamin D.

Calcium:

Calcium is an essential nutrient that is important for bone health. Studies have shown that low levels of calcium can be associated with an increased risk of osteoarthritis and rheumatoid arthritis. Calcium can be found in foods such as dairy products, leafy green vegetables, and fortified foods.

Antioxidants:

Antioxidants are compounds that help protect the body from damage caused by free radicals. Free radicals are molecules that can cause inflammation and damage to cells. Foods that are high in antioxidants, such as fruits and vegetables, can be effective in reducing inflammation and managing arthritis symptoms.

Anti-Inflammatory Foods:

Foods that have anti-inflammatory properties can be effective in reducing joint pain and stiffness in people with arthritis. Examples of anti-inflammatory foods include fatty fish, olive oil, nuts, and whole grains.

Limit Processed Foods:

Processed foods are often high in saturated and trans fats, which can contribute to inflammation in the body. Limiting processed foods and focusing on whole, nutrient-dense foods can be an effective dietary strategy for managing arthritis symptoms.

Hydration:

Staying hydrated is important for overall health and can help reduce inflammation in the body. Drinking plenty of water and other hydrating fluids, such as herbal tea, can be an effective dietary strategy for managing arthritis symptoms.

It is important to note that there is no one-size-fits-all approach to nutrition and diet for arthritis. It is important to work with a healthcare professional to determine the appropriate nutrition and diet strategies for managing arthritis symptoms and improving overall quality of life.

Foods that may help

Arthritis is a chronic condition that can cause pain, stiffness, and inflammation in the joints. While there are several conventional treatments available for managing arthritis symptoms, certain foods may also help alleviate symptoms. Here are some foods that may help manage arthritis:

Fatty Fish:

Fatty fish, such as salmon, tuna, and mackerel, are rich in omega-3 fatty acids. Omega-3 fatty acids have anti-inflammatory properties and can help reduce joint pain and stiffness in people with arthritis. It is recommended to consume at least two servings of fatty fish per week.

Turmeric:

Turmeric is a spice that contains a compound called curcumin, which has anti-inflammatory properties. Studies have shown that turmeric can be effective in reducing joint pain and stiffness in people with osteoarthritis and rheumatoid arthritis. Turmeric can be added to dishes as a spice or taken as a supplement.

Ginger:

Ginger is a root that contains compounds called gingerols and shogaols, which have anti-inflammatory properties. Studies have shown that ginger can be effective in reducing joint pain and stiffness in people with osteoarthritis and rheumatoid arthritis. Ginger can be added to dishes as a spice or taken as a supplement.

Berries:

Berries, such as strawberries, blueberries, and raspberries, are rich in antioxidants. Antioxidants help protect the body from damage caused by free radicals, which can contribute to inflammation and joint damage in people with arthritis. Berries can be consumed fresh or frozen and can be added to smoothies or yogurt.

Broccoli:

Broccoli is a cruciferous vegetable that contains a compound called sulforaphane, which has anti-inflammatory properties. Studies have shown that consuming broccoli can help reduce inflammation in the body and may help manage arthritis symptoms.

Walnuts:

Walnuts are a type of nut that are rich in omega-3 fatty acids and antioxidants. Studies have shown that consuming walnuts can help reduce inflammation in the body and may help manage arthritis symptoms. Walnuts can be added to salads or eaten as a snack.

Olive Oil:

Olive oil is a type of oil that is rich in monounsaturated fatty acids and antioxidants. Studies have shown that consuming olive oil can help reduce inflammation in the body and may help manage arthritis symptoms. Olive oil can be used as a cooking oil or added to salads as a dressing.

It is important to note that there is no one-size-fits-all approach to managing arthritis with diet. It is important to work with a healthcare professional to determine the appropriate dietary strategies for managing arthritis symptoms and improving overall quality of life.

Foods to avoid

Arthritis is a chronic condition that can cause pain, stiffness, and inflammation in the joints. While there are several conventional treatments available for managing arthritis symptoms, certain foods may contribute to inflammation and worsen symptoms. Here are some foods to avoid if you have arthritis:

Processed Foods:

Processed foods, such as packaged snacks, baked goods, and frozen dinners, are often high in saturated and trans fats, which can contribute to inflammation in the body. Processed foods may also be high in added sugars and sodium, which can contribute to weight gain and may exacerbate arthritis symptoms.

Sugary Beverages:

Sugary beverages, such as soda, sports drinks, and fruit juice, are often high in added sugars. Consuming sugary beverages can contribute to weight gain and inflammation in the body, which can exacerbate arthritis symptoms. It is recommended to limit consumption of sugary beverages and opt for water, herbal tea, or unsweetened beverages instead.

Red Meat:

Red meat, such as beef and pork, is high in saturated fats, which can contribute to inflammation in the body. Red meat may also contain compounds that can worsen inflammation in people with arthritis. It is recommended to limit consumption of red meat and opt for lean protein sources, such as chicken, fish, or plant-based protein sources instead.

Fried and Fast Foods:

Fried and fast foods, such as French fries, fried chicken, and burgers, are often high in saturated and trans fats, which can contribute to inflammation in the body. Fried and fast foods may also be high in added sugars and sodium, which can contribute to weight gain and may exacerbate arthritis symptoms. It is recommended to limit consumption of fried and fast foods and opt for whole, nutrient-dense foods instead.

Alcohol:

Alcohol can contribute to inflammation in the body and may exacerbate arthritis symptoms. It is recommended to limit consumption of alcohol or avoid it altogether if you have arthritis.

Dairy Products:

Dairy products, such as milk, cheese, and yogurt, may worsen inflammation in some people with arthritis. Dairy products may contain compounds that can contribute to inflammation in the body. It is recommended to limit consumption of dairy products or opt for low-fat or non-dairy alternatives, such as almond or soy milk, instead.

Nightshade Vegetables:

Nightshade vegetables, such as tomatoes, potatoes, and peppers, contain a compound called solanine, which may contribute to inflammation in some people with arthritis. It is recommended to limit consumption of nightshade vegetables or eliminate them from the diet altogether if you have arthritis.

It is important to note that there is no one-size-fits-all approach to managing arthritis with diet. It is important to work with a healthcare professional to determine the appropriate dietary strategies for managing arthritis symptoms and improving overall quality of life.

Maintaining a healthy weight

Maintaining a healthy weight is important for overall health and can be particularly beneficial for people with arthritis. Arthritis is a chronic condition that can cause pain, stiffness, and inflammation in the joints. Excess weight can place additional stress on the joints and worsen arthritis symptoms. Here are some tips for maintaining a healthy weight if you have arthritis:

Eat a Balanced Diet:

Eating a balanced diet is important for maintaining a healthy weight. A balanced diet should include a variety of fruits, vegetables, lean protein sources, whole grains, and healthy fats. It is important to limit consumption of processed foods, sugary beverages, and foods high in saturated and trans fats.

Control Portion Sizes:

Controlling portion sizes can help manage calorie intake and maintain a healthy weight. It is recommended to use smaller plates and bowls and to measure portions of food to ensure accurate serving sizes.

Stay Hydrated:

Drinking water can help manage appetite and prevent overeating. It is recommended to drink at least eight glasses of water per day.

Be Physically Active:

Regular physical activity can help manage weight and improve arthritis symptoms. Low-impact exercises, such as walking, swimming, and cycling, can be effective in managing weight and improving joint health.

Consider Physical Therapy:

Physical therapy can be helpful for people with arthritis who may have difficulty with exercise or have joint pain that limits physical activity. Physical therapists can develop customized exercise plans that are safe and effective for people with arthritis.

Get Enough Sleep:

Getting enough sleep can help manage appetite and prevent overeating. It is recommended to aim for at least seven to eight hours of sleep per night.

Work with a Healthcare Professional:

Working with a healthcare professional, such as a registered dietitian or a physician, can be helpful in developing a personalized weight management plan. Healthcare professionals can provide guidance on healthy eating habits, physical activity, and weight management strategies.

Maintaining a healthy weight is important for overall health and can be particularly beneficial for people with arthritis. Excess weight can worsen arthritis symptoms and place additional stress on the joints. Eating a balanced diet, controlling portion sizes, staying hydrated, being physically active, considering physical therapy, getting enough sleep, and working with a healthcare professional are all effective strategies for managing weight and improving arthritis symptoms.

Chapter Seven

Exercise and Physical Therapy

Exercise and physical therapy can be effective in managing arthritis symptoms and improving joint health. Arthritis is a chronic condition that can cause pain, stiffness, and inflammation in the joints. Regular exercise and physical therapy can help reduce pain, improve joint mobility, and increase strength and flexibility. Here are some tips for incorporating exercise and physical therapy into your arthritis management plan:

Consult with a Healthcare Professional:

Before starting an exercise or physical therapy program, it is important to consult with a healthcare professional, such as a physician or physical therapist. Healthcare professionals can provide guidance on safe and effective exercise and physical therapy strategies for managing arthritis symptoms.

Choose Low-Impact Activities:

Low-impact activities, such as walking, cycling, and swimming, are effective in managing arthritis symptoms without placing excessive stress on the joints. High-impact activities, such as running and jumping, can worsen arthritis symptoms and should be avoided or limited.

Incorporate Strength Training:

Strength training can help improve joint stability and increase muscle strength. Resistance bands, weights, and bodyweight exercises can be effective in managing arthritis symptoms and improving joint health.

Focus on Flexibility:

Stretching and flexibility exercises can help improve joint mobility and reduce stiffness. Yoga and Pilates are effective in managing arthritis symptoms and improving joint health.

Consider Aquatic Therapy:

Aquatic therapy, or water-based exercise, can be effective in managing arthritis symptoms and improving joint health. The buoyancy of water can reduce stress on the joints, making it an ideal option for people with arthritis.

Practice Good Posture:

Good posture can help reduce stress on the joints and improve joint alignment. Healthcare professionals can provide guidance on proper posture and alignment during exercise and daily activities.

Incorporate Rest and Recovery:

Rest and recovery are important for managing arthritis symptoms and preventing injury. It is important to incorporate rest days into an exercise program and to avoid overexertion.

Work with a Physical Therapist:

Physical therapy can be effective in managing arthritis symptoms and improving joint health. Physical therapists can develop customized exercise and physical therapy plans that are safe and effective for people with arthritis.

The benefits of exercise

Exercise has numerous benefits for overall health and can be particularly beneficial for people with arthritis. Arthritis is a chronic condition that can cause pain, stiffness, and inflammation in the joints. Regular exercise can help reduce pain, improve joint mobility, and increase strength and flexibility. Here are some of the benefits of exercise for people with arthritis:

Reduces Pain:

Regular exercise can help reduce arthritis pain by strengthening the muscles around the joints, improving joint mobility, and reducing inflammation.

Improves Joint Mobility:

Exercise can help improve joint mobility by increasing range of motion and reducing stiffness. This can help people with arthritis maintain independence and perform daily activities more easily.

Increases Strength and Flexibility:

Exercise can help increase muscle strength and flexibility, which can help reduce the stress on joints and improve joint stability.

Reduces Inflammation:

Exercise can help reduce inflammation in the body, which is a common symptom of arthritis. This can help reduce pain and improve overall health.

Improves Cardiovascular Health:

Regular exercise can help improve cardiovascular health by reducing the risk of heart disease, stroke, and other chronic conditions. People with arthritis are at a higher risk for cardiovascular disease, making exercise even more important.

Helps Maintain a Healthy Weight:

Regular exercise can help manage weight and maintain a healthy body mass index (BMI). Excess weight can worsen arthritis symptoms and place additional stress on the joints.

Improves Mental Health:

Exercise has been shown to improve mental health by reducing stress, anxiety, and depression. People with arthritis may experience these conditions at a higher rate than the general population, making exercise an important part of overall mental health.

Promotes Social Interaction:

Exercise can promote social interaction and help people with arthritis connect with others who share similar experiences. This can help reduce feelings of isolation and improve overall quality of life.

Types of exercises for arthritis

Exercise can be an effective strategy for managing arthritis symptoms and improving joint health. There are many types of exercises that can be beneficial for people with arthritis, including low-impact activities, strength training, flexibility exercises, and aquatic therapy. Here are some types of exercises that can be particularly beneficial for people with arthritis:

Low-Impact Activities:

Low-impact activities are effective in managing arthritis symptoms without placing excessive stress on the joints. Walking, cycling, and swimming are all low-impact activities that can help reduce pain, improve joint mobility, and increase strength and flexibility.

Strength Training:

Strength training can help improve joint stability and increase muscle strength. Resistance bands, weights, and bodyweight exercises can be effective in managing arthritis symptoms and improving joint health.

Flexibility Exercises:

Stretching and flexibility exercises can help improve joint mobility and reduce stiffness. Yoga and Pilates are effective in managing arthritis symptoms and improving joint health.

Aquatic Therapy:

Aquatic therapy, or water-based exercise, can be effective in managing arthritis symptoms and improving joint health. The buoyancy of water can reduce stress on the joints, making it an ideal option for people with arthritis.

Tai Chi:

Tai chi is a gentle form of exercise that involves slow, fluid movements. It can be an effective strategy for managing arthritis symptoms and improving joint health. Tai chi can help improve balance, reduce pain, and improve overall well-being.

Cycling:

Cycling is a low-impact activity that can help improve cardiovascular health, reduce pain, and improve joint mobility. It can be an effective strategy for managing arthritis symptoms and improving joint health.

Pilates:

Pilates is a low-impact form of exercise that focuses on strengthening the core muscles and improving posture. It can be an effective strategy for managing arthritis symptoms and improving joint health.

Walking:

Walking is a low-impact activity that can be done anywhere and at any time. It can help improve joint mobility, reduce pain, and improve cardiovascular health.

Working with a physical therapist

Working with a physical therapist can be an effective strategy for managing arthritis symptoms and improving joint health. Physical therapists are trained healthcare professionals who specialize in developing exercise programs to help people with arthritis improve mobility, reduce pain, and increase strength and flexibility. Here are some ways that physical therapy can be beneficial for people with arthritis:

Assessment:

Physical therapists can assess joint mobility, muscle strength, and flexibility to determine the best exercise program for managing arthritis symptoms. They can also evaluate posture and balance to identify potential areas of weakness.

Individualized Exercise Programs:

Physical therapists can develop customized exercise programs that take into account the specific needs of each individual. This can help ensure that the exercise program is safe and effective for managing arthritis symptoms.

Education:

Physical therapists can provide education on proper body mechanics, posture, and movement to help reduce stress on the joints and improve overall joint health. They can also provide information on how to modify activities of daily living to reduce the risk of exacerbating arthritis symptoms.

Manual Therapy:

Physical therapists can use manual therapy techniques, such as massage or joint mobilization, to reduce pain and stiffness in the joints. This can be particularly beneficial for people with arthritis who experience limited mobility or chronic pain.

Aquatic Therapy:

Physical therapists can incorporate aquatic therapy, or water-based exercise, into an exercise program for managing arthritis symptoms. The buoyancy of water can reduce stress on the joints, making it an ideal option for people with arthritis.

Monitoring Progress:

Physical therapists can monitor progress and modify exercise programs as needed to ensure continued improvement in joint health. They can also provide motivation and support to help individuals with arthritis stay committed to their exercise program.

Collaboration with Other Healthcare Professionals:

Physical therapists can work collaboratively with other healthcare professionals, such as rheumatologists or primary care physicians, to develop a comprehensive plan for managing arthritis symptoms.

Chapter Eight

Alternative Therapies

Alternative therapies are becoming increasingly popular for managing arthritis symptoms and improving joint health. While traditional medical treatments, such as medications and physical therapy, can be effective, some people with arthritis may seek out alternative therapies to supplement or replace these treatments. Here are some alternative therapies that have been used for managing arthritis symptoms:

Acupuncture:

Acupuncture is a form of traditional Chinese medicine that involves the insertion of thin needles into specific points on the body. It has been used for managing arthritis symptoms and reducing pain and inflammation.

Massage Therapy:

Massage therapy can help reduce pain and stiffness in the joints, improve circulation, and increase flexibility. Different types of massage, such as Swedish massage or deep tissue massage, may be used depending on the specific needs of each individual.

Chiropractic Care:

Chiropractic care involves manual manipulation of the spine and other joints to reduce pain and improve mobility. It may be used as a complementary therapy for managing arthritis symptoms.

Yoga:

Yoga is a mind-body practice that involves physical postures, breathing exercises, and meditation. It has been shown to reduce pain, improve flexibility, and reduce stress in people with arthritis.

Mindfulness Meditation:

Mindfulness meditation involves focusing attention on the present moment and accepting thoughts and feelings without judgment. It has been shown to reduce stress and improve overall well-being in people with arthritis.

Dietary Supplements:

Dietary supplements, such as glucosamine and chondroitin, have been used for managing arthritis symptoms. While there is some evidence to support their use, the effectiveness of these supplements is still being studied.

Herbal Remedies:

Herbal remedies, such as turmeric or ginger, have been used for managing arthritis symptoms. While there is some evidence to support their use, it is important to consult with a healthcare professional before using herbal remedies to ensure safety and effectiveness.

Heat and Cold Therapy:

Heat and cold therapy can be used to reduce pain and stiffness in the joints. Heat therapy, such as using a heating pad or taking a warm bath, can help improve circulation and reduce muscle tension. Cold therapy, such as using ice packs or taking a cold bath, can help reduce inflammation and swelling.

Acupuncture

Acupuncture is a form of traditional Chinese medicine that has been used for managing arthritis symptoms and reducing pain and inflammation. It involves the insertion of thin needles into specific points on the body, known as acupoints, to stimulate the body's natural healing processes. Here are some ways that acupuncture can be beneficial for people with arthritis:

Pain Reduction:

Acupuncture has been shown to reduce pain in people with arthritis. It works by stimulating the release of endorphins, which are natural pain-relieving chemicals in the body.

Inflammation Reduction:

Acupuncture has been shown to reduce inflammation in people with arthritis. It works by reducing the production of pro-inflammatory cytokines, which are chemicals that contribute to inflammation in the body.

Improved Joint Mobility:

Acupuncture can help improve joint mobility by reducing pain and inflammation in the joints. This can help people with arthritis maintain or improve their ability to perform daily activities.

Stress Reduction:

Acupuncture can help reduce stress in people with arthritis. It works by stimulating the production of neurotransmitters, such as serotonin and dopamine, which are associated with improved mood and reduced stress.

Increased Relaxation:

Acupuncture can help increase relaxation in people with arthritis. It works by stimulating the production of the parasympathetic nervous system, which is responsible for rest and relaxation.

Fewer Side Effects:

Acupuncture is a relatively safe form of treatment with few side effects. This makes it an attractive option for people with arthritis who may be reluctant to use medications with potential side effects.

Massage therapy

Massage therapy is a form of manual therapy that involves the manipulation of the body's soft tissues, such as muscles, tendons, and ligaments. It has been used for managing arthritis symptoms and reducing pain and stiffness in the joints. Here are some ways that massage therapy can be beneficial for people with arthritis:

Pain Reduction:

Massage therapy has been shown to reduce pain in people with arthritis. It works by stimulating the release of endorphins, which are natural pain-relieving chemicals in the body.

Improved Joint Mobility:

Massage therapy can help improve joint mobility by reducing pain and stiffness in the joints. This can help people with arthritis maintain or improve their ability to perform daily activities.

Reduced Inflammation:

Massage therapy can help reduce inflammation in people with arthritis. It works by increasing circulation to the affected areas, which can help reduce inflammation and swelling.

Improved Sleep:

Massage therapy can help improve sleep in people with arthritis. It works by reducing stress and tension in the body, which can help promote relaxation and improve sleep quality.

Reduced Stress and Anxiety:

Massage therapy can help reduce stress and anxiety in people with arthritis. It works by promoting relaxation and reducing muscle tension, which can help improve overall well-being.

Fewer Side Effects:

Massage therapy is a relatively safe form of treatment with few side effects. This makes it an attractive option for people with arthritis who may be reluctant to use medications with potential side effects.

Mind-body practices

Mind-body practices refer to a group of techniques and practices that aim to improve physical health and well-being by promoting the connection between the mind and body. These practices include meditation, yoga, tai chi, and qigong, and have been shown to be effective in managing arthritis symptoms and improving joint health. Here are some ways that mind-body practices can be beneficial for people with arthritis:

Pain Reduction:

Mind-body practices have been shown to reduce pain in people with arthritis. They work by promoting relaxation and reducing stress, which can help reduce pain levels.

Improved Joint Mobility:

Mind-body practices can help improve joint mobility by reducing pain and stiffness in the joints. This can help people with arthritis maintain or improve their ability to perform daily activities.

Reduced Inflammation:

Mind-body practices can help reduce inflammation in people with arthritis. They work by reducing stress levels, which can help reduce the production of pro-inflammatory cytokines, which are chemicals that contribute to inflammation in the body.

Improved Sleep:

Mind-body practices can help improve sleep in people with arthritis. They work by reducing stress and tension in the body, which can help promote relaxation and improve sleep quality.

Reduced Stress and Anxiety:

Mind-body practices can help reduce stress and anxiety in people with arthritis. They work by promoting relaxation and reducing muscle tension, which can help improve overall well-being.

Improved Mood:

Mind-body practices can help improve mood in people with arthritis. They work by promoting relaxation and reducing stress levels, which can help improve mood and reduce symptoms of depression.

Chapter Nine

Assistive Devices and Home Modifications

Assistive devices and home modifications are tools and adaptations that can help people with arthritis perform daily activities with greater ease and independence. These devices and modifications can help reduce pain, improve mobility, and increase safety. Here are some common types of assistive devices and home modifications that can benefit people with arthritis:

Mobility Aids:

Mobility aids, such as canes, walkers, and crutches, can help people with arthritis reduce pain and improve mobility. These aids can help distribute weight off of the affected joint and reduce pressure on the joints.

Braces and Splints:

Braces and splints can help support and stabilize the affected joint, reducing pain and inflammation. These devices can also help improve joint function and reduce the risk of further joint damage.

Ergonomic Tools:

Ergonomic tools, such as specially designed kitchen utensils, can help people with arthritis perform daily tasks with greater ease and less pain. These tools are designed to reduce stress and strain on the joints, making tasks such as cooking and cleaning more manageable.

Home Modifications:

Home modifications, such as installing handrails, grab bars, and wheelchair ramps, can help improve safety and accessibility for people with arthritis. These modifications can help reduce the risk of falls and make it easier to navigate around the home.

Assistive Technology:

Assistive technology, such as voice-activated assistants and smart home devices, can help people with arthritis perform tasks with greater ease and independence. These devices can help reduce the need for manual labor and reduce the strain on the joints.

Choosing the right assistive devices

Choosing the right assistive devices is an important part of managing arthritis symptoms and maintaining independence. With so many options available, it can be overwhelming to decide which device is best suited for individual needs. Here are some factors to consider when choosing the right assistive device:

Type of Arthritis:

Different types of arthritis affect different joints in the body, and therefore require different types of assistive devices. For example, people with osteoarthritis in the knee may benefit from a knee brace, while people with rheumatoid arthritis in the hands may benefit from adaptive kitchen utensils.

Degree of Mobility:

The degree of mobility can also impact the type of assistive device needed. People who require assistance with walking may benefit from a walker or cane, while people who have difficulty standing up from a seated position may benefit from a lift chair.

Size and Weight:

Assistive devices should be appropriate for the individual's size and weight. Choosing a device that is too heavy or too large can cause additional strain on the joints, while choosing a device that is too small or too light may not provide enough support.

Comfort:

Comfort is an important factor to consider when choosing an assistive device. The device should fit comfortably and securely to avoid causing additional pain or discomfort.

Ease of Use:

The device should be easy to use and operate. If the device is too complicated or difficult to use, it may not be effective in improving mobility or reducing pain.

Cost:

Assistive devices can vary in price, and it is important to consider the cost when choosing a device. Some devices may be covered by insurance, while others may require out-of-pocket expenses.

Making your home arthritis-friendly

Arthritis can make daily activities challenging, especially when it comes to navigating around the home. Making your home arthritis-friendly can improve safety and accessibility, and help reduce pain and discomfort. Here are some tips for making your home more arthritis-friendly:

Clear Clutter:

Clearing clutter from your home can help reduce the risk of falls and make it easier to navigate around the home. Remove unnecessary items from walkways, stairs, and other high-traffic areas.

Install Handrails and Grab Bars:

Installing handrails and grab bars can help improve safety and stability when navigating stairs, getting in and out of the bathtub, and using the toilet. These devices can help reduce the risk of falls and provide additional support for people with arthritis.

Improve Lighting:

Improving lighting can help reduce the risk of falls and make it easier to see and navigate around the home. Add additional lighting to dimly lit areas, such as hallways and staircases, and replace burnt-out light bulbs promptly.

Reduce Steps:

Reducing the number of steps required to perform daily activities can help reduce the strain on the joints and make tasks easier to perform. For example, consider installing a handheld showerhead to make it easier to bathe, or using a reacher to grab items from high shelves.

Adapt Your Furniture:

Adapting your furniture can make it easier to get up from a seated position and reduce the strain on the joints. Consider using a lift chair or an adjustable bed to make it easier to get in and out of bed, or using a chair with armrests to provide additional support when sitting down and standing up.

Use Assistive Devices:

Using assistive devices, such as mobility aids, adaptive kitchen utensils, and ergonomic tools, can help reduce the strain on the joints and make daily activities easier to perform. Consult with a healthcare professional or an occupational therapist to determine which assistive devices are best suited for individual needs.

Create a Safe and Accessible Environment:

Creating a safe and accessible environment can help reduce the risk of falls and improve mobility. Consider installing nonslip mats in the bathroom, adding a ramp to the entrance of the home, and using nonskid pads under area rugs.

Adaptive clothing and footwear

People with arthritis often experience joint pain, stiffness, and limited mobility, which can make dressing and footwear choices challenging. Adaptive clothing and footwear are designed to make dressing easier and more comfortable for people with arthritis. Below we will discuss the benefits of adaptive clothing and footwear and provide tips for choosing the right items.

Benefits of Adaptive Clothing

Adaptive clothing is designed with features that make it easier for people with arthritis to dress themselves independently. Some of the benefits of adaptive clothing include:

Ease of Use:

Adaptive clothing is designed with features that make it easier to put on and take off, such as front closures, Velcro, and elastic waistbands. This can reduce the need for bending, twisting, and reaching, which can be challenging for people with arthritis.

Comfort:

Adaptive clothing is designed with soft and breathable fabrics that can help reduce skin irritation and discomfort. The clothing is also designed to fit comfortably over swollen joints and to provide extra room where needed.

Style:

Adaptive clothing is available in a wide range of styles, colors, and patterns, so people with arthritis can choose clothing that suits their personal style and preferences.

Benefits of Adaptive Footwear

Adaptive footwear is designed to provide comfort and support for people with arthritis. Some of the benefits of adaptive footwear include:

Comfort:

Adaptive footwear is designed with features that provide cushioning and support for the feet, which can help reduce pain and discomfort.

Customization:

Adaptive footwear is often designed with removable insoles and inserts that can be customized to provide extra support and cushioning where needed.

Ease of Use:

Adaptive footwear is designed with features that make it easier to put on and take off, such as Velcro straps and slip-on designs. This can reduce the need for bending, twisting, and reaching, which can be challenging for people with arthritis.

Tips for Choosing Adaptive Clothing and Footwear

Choosing the right adaptive clothing and footwear can be a daunting task. Here are some tips to help you make the right choices:

Consult with a Healthcare Professional:

Consulting with a healthcare professional, such as an occupational therapist or a physical therapist, can help you determine which adaptive clothing and footwear are best suited for your individual needs.

Choose Clothing and Footwear with Easy-to-Use Features:

Look for clothing and footwear with easy-to-use features, such as front closures, Velcro, and slip-on designs. These features can make it easier to dress and reduce the need for bending and reaching.

Look for Clothing and Footwear with Soft and Breathable Fabrics:

Choose clothing and footwear made from soft and breathable fabrics that can help reduce skin irritation and discomfort.

Choose Footwear with Good Arch Support:

Look for footwear with good arch support to help distribute weight evenly and reduce pressure on the feet and joints.

Consider Customization Options:

Consider clothing and footwear with customization options, such as removable insoles and inserts, that can be customized to provide extra support and cushioning where needed.

Chapter Ten

Coping with Flares

Flares are a common experience for people living with arthritis. Flares are periods of time when arthritis symptoms, such as joint pain and stiffness, become more intense and widespread. Coping with flares can be challenging, but there are strategies that can help. Below we will discuss what flares are, what triggers flares, and how to cope with flares.

What are Flares?

Flares are periods of time when arthritis symptoms become more intense and widespread. During a flare, people with arthritis may experience increased joint pain, stiffness, fatigue, and difficulty with mobility. Flares can last for a few hours, days, or even weeks, and can be triggered by a variety of factors.

What Triggers Flares?

Flares can be triggered by a variety of factors, including:

Physical Activity:

Overexertion or prolonged physical activity can trigger flares. It is important for people with arthritis to find a balance between staying active and not overdoing it.

Emotional Stress:

Stress and anxiety can trigger flares. It is important for people with arthritis to find ways to manage stress, such as through relaxation techniques or counseling.

Changes in Weather:

Changes in weather, such as changes in temperature and humidity, can trigger flares. It is important for people with arthritis to dress appropriately for the weather and to avoid extreme temperatures.

Infections:

Infections, such as colds and flu, can trigger flares. It is important for people with arthritis to practice good hygiene and to seek medical attention if they suspect they have an infection.

Coping with Flares

Coping with flares can be challenging, but there are strategies that can help. Here are some tips for coping with flares:

Rest:

During a flare, it is important to rest and conserve energy. It may be helpful to take short naps throughout the day or to plan quiet activities that do not require a lot of physical exertion.

Use Heat or Cold Therapy:

Heat therapy, such as taking a warm bath or using a heating pad, can help relieve joint pain and stiffness. Cold therapy, such as using an ice pack, can help reduce inflammation and swelling.

Take Medications as Prescribed:

It is important to take medications as prescribed during a flare. Over-the-counter pain relievers, such as acetaminophen and ibuprofen, may be helpful for mild to moderate pain. Stronger prescription medications, such as nonsteroidal anti-inflammatory drugs (NSAIDs) and corticosteroids, may be needed for more severe symptoms.

Use Assistive Devices:

Assistive devices, such as splints or braces, can help support joints and reduce pain during a flare. Mobility aids, such as canes or walkers, can also help reduce the risk of falls and injury.

Practice Stress Management Techniques:

Stress management techniques, such as deep breathing, meditation, and yoga, can help reduce stress and anxiety during a flare.

Stay Connected:

During a flare, it is important to stay connected with friends, family, and healthcare providers. Talking to others about your symptoms and how you are feeling can help reduce stress and anxiety.

Identifying triggers

Arthritis is a chronic condition that can cause painful inflammation and stiffness in the joints. People with arthritis may experience periods of increased symptoms, known as flares. These flares can be triggered by a variety of factors, including environmental changes, physical activity, and stress. Identifying these triggers can help individuals with arthritis better manage their symptoms and reduce the frequency and severity of flares.

One common trigger for arthritis flares is changes in the weather. Cold and damp weather can make joints feel stiffer and more painful, while warm and dry weather can help alleviate symptoms. This is thought to be due to changes in barometric pressure, which can affect the pressure inside the joints. Paying attention to the weather forecast and planning activities accordingly can help individuals with arthritis avoid triggers related to weather changes.

Physical activity can also trigger arthritis flares. While regular exercise is important for managing arthritis symptoms, overexertion or new activities can cause increased pain and inflammation. Individuals with arthritis should work with their healthcare provider or a physical therapist to develop an exercise plan that is safe and effective for their condition. This may include low-impact activities such as swimming or cycling, and incorporating rest periods into their routine.

Stress is another common trigger for arthritis flares. Stress can cause the body to release hormones that increase inflammation and pain. Practicing stress-reducing activities such as meditation, deep breathing, or yoga may help individuals with arthritis manage their symptoms during periods of increased stress. Additionally, seeking support from family, friends, or a therapist can also help reduce stress and improve overall emotional well-being.

Diet and nutrition may also play a role in triggering arthritis flares. Certain foods, such as those high in sugar or saturated fats, can increase inflammation in the body. On the other hand, a diet rich in anti-inflammatory foods such as fruits, vegetables, and lean protein may help reduce symptoms. Keeping a food diary and noting any changes in symptoms can help individuals with arthritis identify trigger foods and make necessary dietary changes.

Another important aspect of managing arthritis flares is staying on top of medications and following a treatment plan. This may include taking medications as prescribed, attending regular appointments with healthcare providers, and making necessary adjustments to treatment plans as symptoms change. It is important for individuals with arthritis to communicate openly with their healthcare providers about their symptoms and any changes they experience, as this can help inform the most effective treatment plan.

In addition to medical treatments, individuals with arthritis may also benefit from complementary therapies such as massage or acupuncture. These therapies can help reduce pain and inflammation, and improve overall wellbeing. It is important to consult with a healthcare provider before starting any new complementary therapy, as some therapies may interact with medications or worsen symptoms.

Finally, making necessary adjustments to daily activities and the home environment can help reduce the risk of arthritis flares. This may include using assistive devices such as handrails or grab bars, or modifying the home environment to reduce the risk of falls or injuries. Additionally, wearing adaptive clothing or footwear can help reduce strain on the joints and improve overall comfort.

Managing a flare

Managing a flare in arthritis can be challenging, especially when it comes to maintaining your normal routine. Flares can be triggered by a variety of factors such as stress, fatigue, infections, injury, or changes in weather. It is essential to identify the triggers and manage them to reduce the severity of flares.

When it comes to managing a flare, the first step is to listen to your body. It is important to rest and take it easy during a flare. You can plan to take time off work or cancel some appointments to reduce the stress on your joints. Getting adequate sleep is also important during a flare as it helps your body to heal and reduces fatigue.

Applying heat or cold therapy can also help alleviate the pain and discomfort of a flare. Heat therapy, such as using a heating pad or taking a warm bath, can help to relax your muscles and joints, improving blood flow and reducing stiffness. On the other hand, cold therapy, such as using an ice pack or a cold compress, can help to reduce inflammation and numb the pain.

Another effective way to manage a flare is to maintain a healthy and balanced diet. This can help to reduce inflammation and support the immune system, which is essential during a flare. Foods that are high in omega-3 fatty acids, such as salmon, tuna, and flaxseed, are known to have anti-inflammatory properties. Additionally, foods that are high in antioxidants, such as berries, leafy greens, and nuts, can help to protect your body from damage caused by free radicals.

It is also important to stay hydrated during a flare. Drinking enough water and fluids can help to reduce inflammation and improve joint mobility. You can also try drinking herbal teas or warm lemon water to soothe your body and promote relaxation.

Gentle exercises, such as stretching or yoga, can also help to alleviate the symptoms of a flare. However, it is important to consult with your doctor or physical therapist before starting any exercise program during a flare. They can guide you on the best exercises to do and how often to do them to avoid exacerbating the symptoms.

Medications can also be helpful in managing a flare. Over-the-counter pain relievers, such as acetaminophen or nonsteroidal anti-inflammatory drugs (NSAIDs), can help to reduce pain and inflammation. However, it is important to use them as directed and to avoid overusing them to avoid side effects.

If your symptoms are severe or persistent, your doctor may prescribe stronger medications such as corticosteroids or disease-modifying antirheumatic drugs (DMARDs). These medications work to reduce inflammation and slow down the progression of the disease.

Preventing future flares

Arthritis is a chronic condition that causes inflammation and pain in the joints. It can be debilitating and make it difficult for individuals to carry out their daily activities. One of the challenges of living with arthritis is experiencing flares, which can cause sudden and intense pain and inflammation. However, there are ways to prevent future flares and manage the symptoms of arthritis effectively.

The first step in preventing future flares is to identify the triggers that can cause them. Some common triggers of arthritis flares include stress, overexertion, certain foods, changes in weather, and infection. It is essential to keep a journal or note of the activities, foods, or other factors that may have caused a flare-up. This can help to identify the triggers and avoid them in the future.

Managing a flare-up involves reducing inflammation and managing pain. One way to reduce inflammation is by taking nonsteroidal anti-inflammatory drugs (NSAIDs) or disease-modifying antirheumatic drugs (DMARDs) prescribed by a doctor. NSAIDs are over-the-counter pain relievers that can help to reduce inflammation, while DMARDs are medications that help to slow down the progression of arthritis.

Another way to manage pain and inflammation during a flare-up is by applying heat or cold therapy. Cold therapy can help to reduce swelling and inflammation, while heat therapy can help to ease muscle stiffness and joint pain. Heat therapy can be applied through a hot bath, heating pad, or warm towel, while cold therapy can be applied through ice packs or cold compresses.

Physical activity can also help to manage the symptoms of arthritis and prevent future flares. Exercise can help to reduce inflammation, improve joint mobility and flexibility, and build strength in the muscles that support the joints. However, it is important to speak with a healthcare professional before starting an exercise regimen, as certain types of exercise may be more suitable for individuals with arthritis.

In addition to exercise, a healthy diet can also help to prevent future flares. A diet rich in fruits, vegetables, whole grains, and lean proteins can help to reduce inflammation and promote overall health. Avoiding foods that may trigger flares, such as those high in saturated fats and sugar, can also help to prevent future flare-ups.

Finally, it is important to manage stress, as it can be a significant trigger of arthritis flares. Stress can cause inflammation and worsen the symptoms of arthritis. Techniques such as deep breathing, meditation, and yoga can help to reduce stress and improve overall well-being.

Chapter Eleven

Arthritis in the Workplace

Arthritis is a common condition that can affect people of all ages and backgrounds. It is a condition that causes inflammation in the joints, which can lead to pain, stiffness, and limited mobility. Arthritis can have a significant impact on an individual's ability to perform everyday tasks, including those related to work. For this reason, it is important to understand how to manage arthritis in the workplace.

The first step in managing arthritis in the workplace is to understand the condition and how it affects your body. There are many different types of arthritis, each with its own set of symptoms and complications. Some of the most common types of arthritis include osteoarthritis, rheumatoid arthritis, and psoriatic arthritis.

Osteoarthritis is the most common type of arthritis and is often caused by wear and tear on the joints. Rheumatoid arthritis is an autoimmune disorder in which the body's immune system attacks the joints, causing inflammation and damage. Psoriatic arthritis is a type of arthritis that is associated with psoriasis, a skin condition that causes red, scaly patches on the skin.

Once you have a better understanding of your condition, it is important to work with your employer to find ways to manage your arthritis in the workplace. One of the most important things you can do is to create an ergonomic workspace that is designed to reduce the strain on your joints. This might include using a keyboard and mouse that are designed to reduce strain on the hands and wrists, as well as an adjustable chair that provides proper support for your back.

In addition to creating an ergonomic workspace, it is important to take breaks throughout the day to stretch and move your joints. This can help to reduce stiffness and improve your range of motion. You may also want to consider using assistive devices, such as a brace or splint, to help support your joints and reduce pain and swelling.

Another important factor to consider when managing arthritis in the workplace is communication. It is important to talk to your employer and coworkers about your condition and any accommodations that you may need. This might include requesting a flexible work schedule, modified duties, or additional breaks throughout the day.

It is also important to take care of yourself outside of work. This might include following a healthy diet and exercise program, getting enough rest, and managing stress. Stress can exacerbate arthritis symptoms, so it is important to find ways to manage stress, such as practicing relaxation techniques or talking to a therapist.

In some cases, it may be necessary to take time off work to manage your arthritis symptoms. This might include taking sick leave or applying for disability benefits. It is important to talk to your healthcare provider and your employer about your options and to ensure that you have the necessary documentation to support your claims.

Knowing your rights

Arthritis can be a challenging condition to live with, and it can also impact a person's ability to work. However, people with arthritis have rights in the workplace, and knowing these rights can make a big difference in their job satisfaction and overall well-being. Below we will discuss some of the key things to know about workplace rights for people with arthritis.

First and foremost, it's important to understand that arthritis is considered a disability under the Americans with Disabilities Act (ADA). This means that employers are required by law to provide reasonable accommodations to employees with arthritis, as they would for any other disability. Reasonable accommodations are adjustments or modifications to the job or workplace that enable an employee to perform the essential functions of their job.

Examples of reasonable accommodations for people with arthritis might include ergonomic tools or equipment to help with typing or other repetitive tasks, a modified schedule to allow for rest breaks or medical appointments, or a modified workstation to reduce physical strain. It's important to note that the specific accommodations needed will vary depending on the individual's job requirements and the type and severity of their arthritis.

If you have arthritis and you need accommodations in the workplace, the first step is to talk to your employer or human resources representative. Explain your needs and provide any necessary documentation from your healthcare provider to support your request. Your employer is required to engage in an interactive process with you to determine what accommodations are reasonable and feasible. It's important to be open and honest about your needs and to work collaboratively with your employer to find solutions that work for everyone.

It's also worth noting that employers are not allowed to discriminate against employees with arthritis or any other disability. This means that they cannot fire, demote, or refuse to hire someone because of their arthritis. If you feel that you have experienced discrimination in the workplace, you have the right to file a complaint with the Equal Employment Opportunity Commission (EEOC).

In addition to ADA protections, people with arthritis may also be eligible for leave under the Family and Medical Leave Act (FMLA). The FMLA provides eligible employees with up to 12 weeks of unpaid leave per year for a serious health condition, including arthritis. This can be especially helpful for people who need time off for medical appointments, surgery, or other treatments.

To be eligible for FMLA leave, you must have worked for your employer for at least 12 months and have worked at least 1,250 hours during the previous 12 months. You also need to provide your employer with medical certification from your healthcare provider.

It's important to note that while the ADA and FMLA provide important protections for people with arthritis, they do not guarantee job security. If you are unable to perform the essential functions of your job, even with reasonable accommodations, your employer may be within their rights to terminate your employment. However, they are required to engage in an interactive process to determine what accommodations are reasonable and to explore alternative job opportunities within the company, if possible.

In addition to legal protections, there are also steps that people with arthritis can take to manage their condition in the workplace. For example, it may be helpful to take regular breaks to stretch or move around, or to use heat or cold therapy to manage pain and inflammation. People with arthritis may also benefit from using assistive devices or ergonomic tools to reduce strain on the joints.

It's also important to communicate openly with your employer and coworkers about your needs and limitations. While it can be difficult to disclose a medical condition to others, being upfront about your needs can help ensure that you get the support and accommodations you need to perform your job effectively. If you feel comfortable doing so, consider educating your coworkers about arthritis and how it affects you. This can help build empathy and understanding and can also reduce stigma and discrimination.

Requesting accommodations

Arthritis is a chronic condition that affects millions of people worldwide. While it can be challenging to live with arthritis, there are ways to manage symptoms and maintain a high quality of life. For individuals who work, arthritis can pose unique challenges in the workplace. It's important to know that you have rights and can request accommodations to make your work environment more comfortable and manageable. Below we will we'll explore some of the ways that individuals with arthritis can request accommodations in the workplace.

The first step in requesting accommodations is to understand your rights. The Americans with Disabilities Act (ADA) is a federal law that prohibits discrimination based on disability. The ADA applies to private employers with 15 or more employees, as well as to state and local governments. The law defines a disability as a physical or mental impairment that substantially limits one or more major life activities, including working. Arthritis is considered a disability under the ADA, which means that individuals with arthritis are protected by this law.

Once you understand your rights, you can start thinking about the accommodations that might help you in the workplace. Accommodations can take many forms, depending on the nature of your job and your specific needs. Some examples of accommodations for arthritis might include:

1. Ergonomic office equipment: If you spend a lot of time sitting at a desk, ergonomic office equipment such as an adjustable chair or a keyboard tray can help reduce stress on your joints and minimize pain.

2. Flexible work schedule: Arthritis can cause fatigue and pain that may make it difficult to work a traditional 9-5 schedule. A flexible work schedule that allows for breaks or adjustments to your work hours can be helpful.

3. Telecommuting: If commuting to work is a challenge due to arthritis, telecommuting may be a good option. This can allow you to work from home or another location that is more comfortable and less stressful for your joints.

4. Job restructuring: If certain aspects of your job are particularly challenging due to arthritis, job restructuring may be an option. This could involve reassigning certain tasks or modifying your job duties to better accommodate your needs.

5. Assistive technology: There are many types of assistive technology that can be helpful for individuals with arthritis, such as voice recognition software or ergonomic tools for gripping and grasping objects.

Once you have identified the accommodations that might be helpful for you, it's important to communicate with your employer. This can be a difficult conversation, but it's important to be clear about your needs and how accommodations can help you perform your job more effectively. Your employer may ask for documentation from your doctor or other medical professionals to support your request for accommodations.

It's also important to note that employers are not required to provide every accommodation that is requested. However, they are required to engage in a dialogue with the employee to explore potential accommodations and identify those that are reasonable and effective.

It's important to remember that requesting accommodations is not a sign of weakness or a lack of capability. Rather, it's a way to ensure that you can perform your job to the best of your ability while managing the symptoms of arthritis. It's also important to note that accommodations can benefit not only the individual with arthritis, but the employer as well. When employees are comfortable and able to work to the best of their ability, they are more productive and engaged in their work.

Balancing work and self-care

Living with arthritis can be challenging, especially when it comes to balancing work and self-care. Arthritis is a chronic condition that can cause pain, stiffness, and inflammation in the joints, which can make it difficult to perform daily activities. However, with the right strategies, it is possible to manage arthritis symptoms and maintain a healthy work-life balance.

One of the most important things to keep in mind when managing arthritis is to prioritize self-care. This means taking time to rest and recharge when needed, eating a healthy diet, and engaging in regular exercise. It also means seeking medical treatment when necessary and taking medications as prescribed by a doctor.

In terms of work, it is important to communicate with employers and coworkers about your condition and any accommodations that may be needed. This can include things like ergonomic office equipment, flexible work hours, or modified job duties. By being open and honest about your needs, you can work together to create a more supportive work environment.

Another important aspect of balancing work and self-care with arthritis is learning to manage your time effectively. This can involve planning ahead, prioritizing tasks, and taking breaks when needed. It may also involve learning to say no to additional responsibilities when you are feeling overwhelmed or experiencing a flare-up of symptoms.

In addition to these strategies, there are a number of other tools and resources available to help individuals with arthritis balance work and self-care. These may include support groups, online resources, and apps designed specifically for arthritis management.

One of the keys to successfully balancing work and self-care with arthritis is to be proactive about your health. This means staying informed about your condition and learning as much as you can about effective management strategies. It also means working closely with your doctor to develop a personalized treatment plan that takes into account your specific needs and lifestyle.

Finally, it is important to remember that managing arthritis is an ongoing process. While there may be times when symptoms are more severe or difficult to manage, there will also be times when they are less of a concern. By remaining patient, persistent, and dedicated to your health and well-being, you can successfully balance work and self-care with arthritis and live a fulfilling life.

Chapter Twelve

Relationships and Support

Arthritis can be a challenging condition to live with, and having a support system in place can make a significant difference in managing the physical and emotional aspects of the disease. Relationships with friends, family, and healthcare providers can all play an essential role in providing support and assistance for those living with arthritis.

One of the most important relationships for individuals with arthritis is their healthcare provider. This includes rheumatologists, primary care physicians, physical therapists, and other healthcare professionals. These providers can offer medical advice, prescribe medications, and recommend treatments to help manage arthritis symptoms. It is crucial to establish a good rapport with healthcare providers, to ask questions, and to discuss concerns about arthritis symptoms and management.

Family and friends can also play a crucial role in providing support for those with arthritis. For instance, loved ones can provide emotional support, assist with household tasks, and help with transportation to medical appointments. Friends and family members can also offer a listening ear and help individuals with arthritis stay engaged in activities they enjoy.

Support groups can also be an essential source of support for those with arthritis. These groups provide individuals with a chance to connect with others who share similar experiences and challenges. Support groups can offer emotional support, practical advice, and opportunities to participate in activities and events with others.

In addition to traditional support groups, online communities and social media groups can also provide a source of support for individuals with arthritis. These communities allow individuals to connect with others from around the world, share their experiences, and offer support and advice.

It is important to remember that living with arthritis can be emotionally challenging, and it is not uncommon to experience feelings of anxiety, depression, or frustration. Seeking support from a therapist or counselor can be helpful in managing these emotions and finding coping strategies to manage the emotional impact of arthritis.

Self-care is also an essential aspect of managing arthritis and can help individuals maintain a sense of control and independence. This may include engaging in physical activity, eating a balanced diet, and getting adequate rest. Self-care can also involve managing stress through activities such as meditation, yoga, or deep breathing exercises.

For individuals with arthritis, it can be helpful to communicate their needs and limitations to others. This may involve explaining the impact of arthritis on daily activities or discussing any necessary accommodations needed in the workplace. By openly communicating with others, individuals with arthritis can work to establish supportive relationships and find ways to manage their condition more effectively.

Communicating with loved ones

Arthritis can have a significant impact on a person's relationships, and communicating with loved ones about the condition is an essential part of managing it. Arthritis is a chronic condition that can cause pain, stiffness, and swelling in the joints, making it difficult for a person to perform daily activities. This can cause frustration and stress, not just for the person with arthritis, but also for their loved ones.

One of the most important things to remember when communicating with loved ones about arthritis is to be open and honest. It is important to share your experiences with them and let them know how you are feeling. This can help them understand what you are going through and what they can do to support you.

It is also important to be specific about the kind of help and support you need. For example, you might need help with household chores or assistance with transportation to medical appointments. Letting your loved ones know how they can help you can make them feel useful and valued, while also making your life easier.

It is also important to be realistic about your limitations. Arthritis can make it difficult to perform certain tasks or participate in certain activities. Letting your loved ones know what you can and cannot do can help prevent misunderstandings and frustration.

Another important aspect of communicating with loved ones about arthritis is to educate them about the condition. Many people do not understand the impact that arthritis can have on a person's life. Educating them about the symptoms, causes, and treatment options can help them understand what you are going through and how they can support you.

In addition to communicating with loved ones, it is also important to seek out support from others who are dealing with similar challenges. This can be done through support groups, online forums, or social media. Connecting with others who understand what you are going through can provide emotional support and valuable information about managing the condition.

It is also important to seek professional help if needed. This may include working with a therapist or counselor to help manage the emotional toll of living with a chronic condition. It may also involve working with a physical therapist or occupational therapist to learn techniques for managing pain and stiffness.

In addition to seeking professional help, there are also many self-care techniques that can be helpful in managing arthritis. This may include regular exercise, a healthy diet, stress management techniques, and getting enough sleep. These techniques can help manage the symptoms of arthritis and improve overall quality of life.

Finding a support group

Living with arthritis can be challenging, and it is often helpful to have a support system in place. One way to find support is by joining a support group. Support groups provide a space for individuals with arthritis to connect, share experiences, and learn from one another.

There are many different types of arthritis support groups available, both in-person and online. Some are run by organizations such as the Arthritis Foundation or local hospitals, while others are led by individuals who have personal experience with arthritis. Some support groups are focused on a specific type of arthritis, while others are open to anyone with any type of arthritis.

There are many benefits to joining an arthritis support group. Here are a few:

1. Connection: Living with arthritis can be isolating, and it can be comforting to connect with others who are going through similar experiences.

2. Education: Support groups can be a great source of information about arthritis, treatments, and coping strategies.

3. Emotional support: Arthritis can be emotionally challenging, and support groups provide a safe space to share feelings and receive support.

4. Empowerment: By connecting with others who have arthritis, individuals can feel empowered and inspired to take control of their health and well-being.

If you are interested in joining an arthritis support group, here are some steps you can take:

5. Ask your healthcare provider: Your healthcare provider may be able to recommend a support group in your area.

6. Check with arthritis organizations: Organizations such as the Arthritis Foundation may have information about support groups in your area.

7. Search online: Many support groups have an online presence, and a quick internet search may lead you to a group that fits your needs.

8. Attend meetings: Once you have found a support group, attend a meeting to see if it is a good fit for you.

It is important to remember that not all support groups are the same, and what works for one person may not work for another. It may take some time to find the right group for you, but it can be worth the effort.

In addition to traditional support groups, there are also online communities that can provide support and connection. These can be especially helpful for individuals who have limited mobility or live in remote areas. Online communities may take the form of forums, chat rooms, or social media groups. It is important to be cautious when joining online communities and to ensure that the group is reputable and safe.

Building a healthcare team

Arthritis is a chronic condition that requires ongoing management and treatment. Building a healthcare team is an essential part of managing arthritis. A healthcare team can include various medical professionals, such as primary care physicians, rheumatologists, physical therapists, occupational therapists, and pain management specialists. It is essential to have a team of healthcare professionals to help individuals with arthritis manage their condition and improve their overall health and well-being.

The first step in building a healthcare team is to find a primary care physician who can help manage arthritis symptoms. Primary care physicians can provide referrals to specialists and help monitor medication use. They can also coordinate care between different specialists and provide ongoing support and guidance.

Rheumatologists are specialists who focus on the diagnosis and treatment of arthritis and related conditions. They can help develop a treatment plan and monitor disease progression. Rheumatologists can also recommend lifestyle changes and prescribe medications to manage symptoms.

Physical therapists and occupational therapists are also essential members of a healthcare team. Physical therapists can help individuals with arthritis improve their range of motion, strength, and flexibility. They can also recommend exercises and stretches to reduce pain and improve mobility. Occupational therapists can help individuals with arthritis modify their daily activities to reduce pain and improve function. They can also recommend assistive devices and equipment to help with daily tasks.

Pain management specialists can also be part of a healthcare team. These specialists can provide medications and therapies to help manage pain associated with arthritis. They can also recommend alternative therapies, such as acupuncture or massage therapy, to help reduce pain and improve overall well-being.

When building a healthcare team, it is also essential to consider mental health professionals. Arthritis can take a toll on an individual's mental health, leading to depression, anxiety, and stress. Mental health professionals, such as counselors or psychologists, can provide support and guidance to individuals with arthritis and help them cope with the emotional toll of their condition.

Family members and friends can also play an essential role in an individual's healthcare team. They can provide emotional support and help with daily tasks when needed. It is important to communicate with loved ones about the challenges of living with arthritis and let them know how they can best support the individual with the condition.

In addition to healthcare professionals and loved ones, online support groups can also be a valuable resource for individuals with arthritis. Online support groups provide a platform for individuals with similar experiences to connect and share their struggles and successes. They can offer emotional support, practical advice, and encouragement, helping individuals with arthritis feel less isolated and more empowered.

Chapter Thirteen

Managing Arthritis in Children

Arthritis is often associated with older adults, but it can affect people of all ages, including children. Childhood arthritis, also known as juvenile arthritis, is a broad term used to describe several different types of arthritis that affect children under the age of 16. While the exact causes of childhood arthritis are still unknown, it is believed to be an autoimmune disorder that causes the immune system to mistakenly attack healthy joint tissues, resulting in joint inflammation and pain. Below we will discuss the different types of childhood arthritis, their symptoms, and treatment options.

Types of Childhood Arthritis

There are several types of childhood arthritis, with the most common being juvenile idiopathic arthritis (JIA), also known as juvenile rheumatoid arthritis. JIA is a group of chronic arthritis conditions that affect children and can cause joint inflammation, pain, stiffness, and loss of joint function. The subtypes of JIA include oligoarticular, polyarticular, systemic, enthesitis-related, and psoriatic arthritis.

Oligoarticular JIA is the most common subtype of JIA, accounting for 50% of cases. It affects four or fewer joints and often presents in young girls. Polyarticular JIA, on the other hand, affects five or more joints and can present in both girls and boys. Systemic JIA is a rare subtype that can affect multiple joints, as well as other organs, such as the liver, spleen, and lymph nodes. Enthesitis-related JIA is characterized by inflammation in the entheses, which are the points where tendons or ligaments attach to the bones. This type of arthritis often affects the lower extremities, such as the hips, knees, and ankles. Finally, psoriatic arthritis is a subtype of JIA that affects children who also have psoriasis, a skin condition.

Symptoms of Childhood Arthritis

The symptoms of childhood arthritis can vary depending on the type of arthritis and the child's age. Common symptoms include joint pain, stiffness, swelling, and warmth. In some cases, the child may also experience fever, rash, and weight loss. If left untreated, childhood arthritis can lead to joint damage, growth problems, and deformities. It is important to see a doctor if you suspect your child has arthritis, as early diagnosis and treatment can help prevent these complications.

Treatment of Childhood Arthritis

The treatment of childhood arthritis aims to reduce inflammation, relieve pain, and prevent joint damage. The treatment plan will depend on the type of arthritis and the severity of the symptoms. Nonsteroidal anti-inflammatory drugs (NSAIDs) are often used to reduce pain and inflammation. In more severe cases, disease-modifying antirheumatic drugs (DMARDs) may be prescribed to slow down the progression of the disease and protect the joints from damage. Biologic agents, such as tumor necrosis factor inhibitors, may also be used in some cases.

Physical therapy is an essential part of the treatment plan for childhood arthritis. It can help improve joint mobility and reduce pain and stiffness. Exercises that focus on range of motion, strengthening, and aerobic conditioning are usually recommended. In some cases, splints or braces may be used to support the joints and reduce pain.

In addition to medication and physical therapy, lifestyle modifications can also help manage childhood arthritis symptoms. Maintaining a healthy weight, eating a balanced diet, and getting enough rest are all important for managing arthritis symptoms. Stress reduction techniques, such as mindfulness meditation and yoga, can also be beneficial.

Recognizing the signs

Arthritis is often thought of as a disease that affects older individuals, but it can also affect children. Juvenile idiopathic arthritis (JIA) is the most common type of arthritis in children, affecting approximately 300,000 children in the United States. It is a chronic autoimmune disease that can cause joint inflammation and pain, and can affect a child's growth and development. As with any condition, recognizing the signs and symptoms of JIA is important for early diagnosis and treatment.

The signs and symptoms of JIA can vary widely from child to child, and can even vary within the same child over time. The most common symptom is joint pain, which may be accompanied by swelling and stiffness. Children may also experience a decreased range of motion in affected joints, as well as fatigue and malaise. In some cases, JIA can cause eye inflammation, which can lead to vision problems if left untreated.

It is important to note that joint pain and stiffness are not always signs of JIA. Many children experience these symptoms at some point during their development, and most do not have arthritis. However, if a child experiences persistent joint pain, swelling, or stiffness, it is important to seek medical attention. Other signs that may indicate JIA include a limp, reluctance to use a limb, or unexplained fever.

Diagnosing JIA can be challenging, as there is no single test that can definitively diagnose the condition. Instead, doctors will typically perform a physical exam, order blood tests, and may perform imaging tests such as X-rays or MRIs. They will also ask about the child's medical history and family history, as JIA is believed to have a genetic component.

Once a diagnosis of JIA has been made, treatment can begin. The goal of treatment is to manage symptoms, reduce inflammation, and prevent long-term joint damage. There are a variety of treatment options available, depending on the type and severity of the child's JIA.

Nonsteroidal anti-inflammatory drugs (NSAIDs) are often used to manage pain and inflammation in children with JIA. In some cases, disease-modifying antirheumatic drugs (DMARDs) may be prescribed to slow the progression of the disease and prevent joint damage. Biologic drugs, which target specific components of the immune system, may also be used in some cases.

Physical therapy and regular exercise can also be helpful in managing JIA. A physical therapist can work with the child to develop a customized exercise program that can help improve joint mobility and reduce pain and stiffness. In addition, assistive devices such as braces or splints may be recommended to help support affected joints.

Managing JIA can be a complex and ongoing process, and it is important for children with the condition to receive ongoing medical care and support. In addition to working with a healthcare team that includes a pediatric rheumatologist and other specialists, children with JIA may also benefit from connecting with support groups or other resources for families affected by arthritis.

Treatment options

Arthritis is a condition that affects people of all ages, including children. Children with arthritis may experience pain, swelling, stiffness, and difficulty with movement, all of which can have a significant impact on their quality of life. Fortunately, there are many treatment options available that can help manage the symptoms of arthritis in children and improve their overall well-being.

The treatment options for arthritis in children depend on the type and severity of the condition. In some cases, medications may be prescribed to reduce pain and inflammation. Nonsteroidal anti-inflammatory drugs (NSAIDs) are commonly used to treat arthritis in children, as they can help reduce pain and inflammation. However, they should be used with caution, as they can cause stomach upset, bleeding, and kidney damage if taken for prolonged periods of time.

Corticosteroids may also be used to treat arthritis in children. These medications work by reducing inflammation in the body, but they can have significant side effects, including weight gain, high blood pressure, and bone loss. As a result, they are usually only used for short periods of time and under close medical supervision.

Disease-modifying antirheumatic drugs (DMARDs) may also be used to treat arthritis in children. These medications work by suppressing the immune system, which can help reduce inflammation and prevent joint damage. However, they can have serious side effects, including an increased risk of infection and liver damage, so they are usually only used in severe cases or when other treatments have not been effective.

In addition to medications, physical therapy can also be an effective treatment for arthritis in children. Physical therapy can help improve joint mobility, reduce pain and stiffness, and increase strength and flexibility. A physical therapist can work with children to develop an exercise program that is tailored to their specific needs and abilities.

Occupational therapy may also be recommended for children with arthritis. Occupational therapists can help children learn new ways to perform daily activities, such as getting dressed, brushing their teeth, and using utensils, that may have become difficult due to arthritis. They can also recommend assistive devices, such as splints or braces, to help support affected joints and improve mobility.

In some cases, surgery may be necessary to treat arthritis in children. Joint replacement surgery may be recommended if the arthritis has caused significant joint damage and is affecting the child's quality of life. However, this is usually only considered as a last resort when other treatments have not been effective.

It is important for children with arthritis to receive ongoing care and monitoring from a healthcare team, which may include a rheumatologist, a pediatrician, a physical therapist, an occupational therapist, and a psychologist or social worker. The healthcare team can work together to develop a comprehensive treatment plan that addresses the child's physical, emotional, and social needs.

In addition to medical treatment, there are many lifestyle changes that can help manage the symptoms of arthritis in children. Eating a healthy diet that is rich in fruits, vegetables, and whole grains can help reduce inflammation in the body. Regular exercise, such as swimming or cycling, can also help improve joint mobility and reduce pain and stiffness.

It is important for children with arthritis to get plenty of rest and avoid activities that put too much stress on their joints. Parents and caregivers can also help children with arthritis by providing emotional support, encouraging independence, and helping them cope with the challenges of living with a chronic condition.

Supporting your child's emotional wellbeing

Arthritis is a condition that affects people of all ages, including children. It can be difficult for a child to cope with the pain and limitations caused by arthritis, and it can also have an impact on their emotional wellbeing. As a parent or caregiver, it is important to not only address the physical symptoms of arthritis but also to support your child's emotional needs.

One of the first steps in supporting your child's emotional wellbeing is to understand how arthritis can affect their mental health. Children with arthritis may feel frustrated, anxious, or even depressed because of the pain and limitations caused by their condition. They may feel left out of activities or social events because of their symptoms, which can lead to feelings of isolation and loneliness. It is important to acknowledge these feelings and provide a safe and supportive environment for your child to express them.

Another way to support your child's emotional wellbeing is to encourage them to talk about their condition. Children may feel embarrassed or shy about their arthritis, especially if they are the only child in their class or peer group with the condition. However, talking openly about their experiences can help them feel less alone and more understood. Encourage your child to share their feelings with you, their doctor, and other trusted adults in their life.

In addition to emotional support, there are also practical steps you can take to help your child manage their arthritis. This may include working with a physical therapist to develop an exercise plan that is safe and effective for their condition. Physical activity can not only help manage arthritis symptoms but also promote positive mental health by reducing stress and improving mood.

Another important aspect of managing arthritis in children is medication management. Your child's doctor may prescribe medications to manage pain and inflammation associated with arthritis. It is important to follow their instructions carefully and monitor your child for any side effects or changes in symptoms.

In some cases, surgery may be necessary to manage arthritis in children. This can be a difficult and scary experience for a child, so it is important to provide emotional support and reassurance throughout the process. Encourage your child to ask questions and express their feelings about the surgery and recovery process.

Finally, it is important to encourage your child to engage in activities that they enjoy and find fulfilling. This may include hobbies, sports, or other extracurricular activities. While it may require some adaptation to accommodate their arthritis, it is important for your child to continue to pursue their interests and passions. This can help promote positive self-esteem and emotional wellbeing.

Chapter Fourteen

Aging and Arthritis

Arthritis is a common condition that affects people of all ages, but it is more prevalent in older adults. It is estimated that over 50% of people aged 65 and older have arthritis. While arthritis is often associated with pain and stiffness in the joints, it can also have a significant impact on an older person's quality of life. Below we will explore the impact of aging on arthritis, the types of arthritis that are most common in older adults, and the treatment options available.

As people age, their bodies undergo various changes, including a loss of bone density, muscle mass, and joint flexibility. These changes can make older adults more vulnerable to arthritis, as well as other musculoskeletal conditions. Additionally, older adults are more likely to have other chronic health conditions, such as diabetes, heart disease, and obesity, which can exacerbate the symptoms of arthritis.

The two most common types of arthritis in older adults are osteoarthritis (OA) and rheumatoid arthritis (RA). Osteoarthritis is a degenerative joint disease that occurs when the cartilage that cushions the joints breaks down over time, causing pain, stiffness, and swelling. Osteoarthritis is most common in the hips, knees, and hands. Rheumatoid arthritis, on the other hand, is an autoimmune disease that causes inflammation in the joints, which can lead to pain, swelling, and deformity. Rheumatoid arthritis is most common in the hands, feet, and wrists.

In addition to osteoarthritis and rheumatoid arthritis, older adults may also be at risk for other forms of arthritis, such as gout, psoriatic arthritis, and septic arthritis. Gout is a type of arthritis that occurs when uric acid crystals build up in the joints, causing intense pain and inflammation. Psoriatic arthritis is a type of arthritis that occurs in people with psoriasis, a skin condition that causes red, scaly patches. Septic arthritis is a type of arthritis that occurs when a joint becomes infected.

Treatment options for arthritis in older adults vary depending on the type and severity of the condition. For osteoarthritis, treatments may include over-the-counter pain relievers, such as acetaminophen or nonsteroidal anti-inflammatory drugs (NSAIDs), physical therapy, and lifestyle modifications, such as weight loss and exercise. In some cases, joint replacement surgery may be necessary.

For rheumatoid arthritis and other forms of inflammatory arthritis, treatments may include disease-modifying antirheumatic drugs (DMARDs), biologics, and corticosteroids. These medications can help reduce inflammation, slow joint damage, and improve quality of life. Other treatments for arthritis may include heat or cold therapy, massage, and acupuncture.

In addition to medical treatments, there are several things that older adults with arthritis can do to manage their symptoms and improve their quality of life. These may include maintaining a healthy weight, engaging in regular exercise, eating a healthy diet rich in fruits, vegetables, and whole grains, and getting enough rest and sleep. Older adults may also benefit from assistive devices, such as canes, walkers, and mobility scooters, to help them stay mobile and independent.

Arthritis can also have a significant impact on an older adult's emotional wellbeing. Chronic pain and limitations in mobility can lead to feelings of frustration, depression, and anxiety. It is important for older adults with arthritis to seek emotional support from loved ones, join support groups, and engage in activities that bring them joy and fulfillment.

The impact of age on arthritis

Arthritis is a condition that affects people of all ages, but it is more common in older adults. Age is one of the major risk factors for developing arthritis, with the likelihood of developing the condition increasing as a person gets older. Below we will explore the impact of age on arthritis, including the causes, symptoms, and treatment options.

As a person ages, the risk of developing arthritis increases due to a variety of factors. These include wear and tear on the joints over time, changes in the immune system, and the accumulation of other medical conditions. Osteoarthritis is the most common form of arthritis in older adults, and it is caused by the wear and tear of the cartilage that cushions the joints. As this cartilage wears down, the bones may rub against each other, causing pain, stiffness, and inflammation.

In addition to osteoarthritis, older adults may also be at increased risk for other types of arthritis, including rheumatoid arthritis, gout, and psoriatic arthritis. Rheumatoid arthritis is an autoimmune disease that can affect people of any age, but it is more common in older adults. Gout is a type of arthritis caused by the buildup of uric acid crystals in the joints, and it is more common in men over the age of 40. Psoriatic arthritis is a type of arthritis that can develop in people with psoriasis, and it is more common in adults over the age of 30.

Symptoms of arthritis in older adults can be similar to those experienced by younger people with the condition, but there are some differences. Older adults may experience more severe pain and stiffness in their joints, as well as more difficulty with mobility and daily activities. They may also be more likely to have other medical conditions that can make arthritis symptoms worse, such as heart disease, diabetes, and obesity.

Treatment options for arthritis in older adults are similar to those for younger people, but there are some considerations specific to this population. For example, older adults may be more likely to have side effects from medications used to treat arthritis, such as nonsteroidal anti-inflammatory drugs (NSAIDs) and disease-modifying antirheumatic drugs (DMARDs). They may also need to take other medications for other medical conditions, which can interact with arthritis medications.

In addition to medication, older adults with arthritis may benefit from physical therapy and exercise programs designed to improve mobility and range of motion. These programs can also help to strengthen muscles and reduce the risk of falls, which is a major concern for older adults with arthritis. Assistive devices such as canes, walkers, and splints may also be helpful for some older adults with arthritis.

Emotional support is also important for older adults with arthritis, as the condition can be challenging to manage and can impact daily activities and quality of life. Support from family members, friends, and healthcare providers can help older adults with arthritis to cope with their condition and stay engaged in their daily lives.

Strategies for managing arthritis in older adults

Arthritis is a common condition that affects people of all ages, but it is more prevalent in older adults. As we age, the risk of developing arthritis increases, and the condition can have a significant impact on our quality of life. However, there are several strategies that can help manage arthritis in older adults and improve their overall well-being.

One of the most important strategies for managing arthritis in older adults is to stay active. Regular exercise can help reduce joint pain, increase range of motion, and improve overall fitness. Exercise also helps to maintain healthy body weight, which can reduce stress on the joints. Older adults should aim for at least 150 minutes of moderate-intensity exercise per week, such as walking, cycling, or swimming. It is important to work with a healthcare provider to develop an appropriate exercise program that takes into account any physical limitations or medical conditions.

Another strategy for managing arthritis in older adults is to eat a healthy diet. A diet rich in fruits, vegetables, whole grains, and lean proteins can help reduce inflammation and promote overall health. Older adults should aim to limit their intake of processed foods, sugary drinks, and saturated fats, which can increase inflammation and contribute to weight gain.

In addition to exercise and diet, there are several other strategies that can help manage arthritis in older adults. These include:

1. Physical therapy: A physical therapist can help develop an individualized exercise program that is safe and effective for older adults with arthritis. They can also teach exercises to improve flexibility, strength, and balance, which can help reduce the risk of falls.

2. Assistive devices: Older adults with arthritis may benefit from using assistive devices such as canes, walkers, or grab bars. These devices can help reduce the stress on the joints and make daily activities easier to perform.

3. Medications: There are several medications available to help manage arthritis in older adults, including nonsteroidal anti-inflammatory drugs (NSAIDs), corticosteroids, and disease-modifying antirheumatic drugs (DMARDs). Older adults should work closely with their healthcare provider to determine the best medication regimen for their individual needs.

4. Surgery: In some cases, surgery may be necessary to treat severe arthritis in older adults. Joint replacement surgery, such as hip or knee replacement, can help improve mobility and reduce pain.

It is also important for older adults with arthritis to manage their emotional well-being. Chronic pain can have a significant impact on mental health, leading to depression, anxiety, and social isolation. Older adults should seek support from family and friends, and consider joining a support group or seeking professional counseling if necessary.

Staying active and engaged

As people age, arthritis becomes increasingly common, affecting their mobility and overall quality of life. Arthritis is a chronic inflammatory disorder that can cause joint pain, swelling, and stiffness. It is most commonly associated with aging and often occurs in older adults. However, the condition can also affect younger people.

Staying active and engaged is essential for seniors with arthritis. This can help maintain joint flexibility, reduce inflammation, and improve overall health and wellbeing. Fortunately, there are numerous strategies that can help older adults manage their arthritis symptoms and continue to enjoy an active and fulfilling life.

One of the most important strategies for managing arthritis in older adults is to maintain an active lifestyle. Regular exercise can help reduce pain and stiffness, increase joint flexibility, and improve overall physical function. Low-impact exercises such as walking, swimming, and cycling are recommended for seniors with arthritis, as they are less likely to cause joint pain and injury.

It is also important for seniors with arthritis to engage in activities that they enjoy and that provide a sense of purpose and fulfillment. This can include hobbies, volunteering, or spending time with family and friends. Engaging in meaningful activities can help reduce stress, improve mood, and enhance overall wellbeing.

In addition to staying active, seniors with arthritis should also focus on maintaining a healthy diet. Eating a balanced diet rich in fruits, vegetables, lean protein, and whole grains can help reduce inflammation and improve overall health. Foods that are high in omega-3 fatty acids, such as fish and nuts, are particularly beneficial for people with arthritis.

In some cases, medications may be necessary to manage arthritis symptoms in older adults. Nonsteroidal anti-inflammatory drugs (NSAIDs) and disease-modifying antirheumatic drugs (DMARDs) are commonly prescribed to reduce pain and inflammation. However, it is important to work closely with a healthcare provider to ensure that medications are being used safely and effectively.

Seniors with arthritis may also benefit from using assistive devices and making modifications to their home environment. This can include using canes or walkers to help with mobility, installing handrails and grab bars in the bathroom, and using cushioned chairs to reduce pressure on the joints.

In addition to physical strategies, it is also important for seniors with arthritis to focus on their emotional wellbeing. Arthritis can be a challenging and isolating condition, and seniors may benefit from joining a support group or seeking counseling. This can provide them with a sense of community and help them manage the emotional impact of their condition.

Chapter Fifteen

Surgery and Joint Replacement

Arthritis is a degenerative condition that causes inflammation in the joints, leading to pain, stiffness, and decreased range of motion. While there are several treatment options available, surgery and joint replacement are often considered when other treatments are no longer effective. Below we will explore the types of surgery and joint replacement procedures available, when they are recommended, and what to expect during and after the procedures.

There are several types of surgeries available for arthritis, including arthroscopy, synovectomy, and osteotomy. Arthroscopy is a minimally invasive surgery that involves the insertion of a small camera into the joint to view and repair damage. This procedure is most commonly used for knees and shoulders and can be done as an outpatient procedure, with minimal scarring and a short recovery time.

Synovectomy involves the removal of the synovial membrane, which lines the joints and can become inflamed and damaged in arthritis. This surgery can help reduce inflammation and pain in the joint, and is commonly performed in the wrists, knees, and hips.

Osteotomy is a procedure that involves the reshaping or removal of bone to correct deformities caused by arthritis. This surgery is often recommended for people with early-stage arthritis who have bone damage or deformities that cannot be corrected by other treatments.

When other treatments are no longer effective, joint replacement surgery may be recommended. Joint replacement involves the removal of the damaged joint and the insertion of an artificial joint made of metal and plastic. The most common joints that are replaced are the knee, hip, and shoulder.

The decision to undergo joint replacement surgery is usually made when other treatments, such as medication and physical therapy, have failed to provide relief. The surgery is typically recommended for people with severe pain, stiffness, and limited mobility that affects their quality of life.

Before the surgery, the patient will undergo a thorough medical evaluation to determine if they are a good candidate for the procedure. This evaluation will include a physical exam, X-rays, and blood tests. The patient will also meet with a physical therapist to discuss pre- and post-operative exercises and rehabilitation.

During the surgery, the patient will be given anesthesia to ensure that they are comfortable and do not feel any pain. The surgeon will make an incision in the affected joint and remove the damaged joint components. The artificial joint will then be inserted and secured in place.

Following the surgery, the patient will stay in the hospital for a few days to monitor their recovery. Physical therapy will begin soon after the surgery to help the patient regain strength and range of motion. The patient will also be given pain medication and antibiotics to prevent infection.

It is important to note that joint replacement surgery is not without risks. While it is generally considered safe, there are risks associated with any surgery, including infection, bleeding, and blood clots. It is important for patients to discuss these risks with their doctor before deciding to undergo surgery.

In addition to surgery and joint replacement, there are several other treatments available for arthritis, including medication, physical therapy, and lifestyle changes. It is important for people with arthritis to work closely with their healthcare team to develop a comprehensive treatment plan that meets their individual needs.

When to consider surgery

Arthritis is a condition that affects millions of people around the world, causing pain, stiffness, and swelling in the joints. While many people are able to manage their symptoms with medication, physical therapy, and other non-surgical treatments, some may eventually require surgery to alleviate their pain and improve their quality of life.

When it comes to considering surgery for arthritis, there are a few key factors to consider. Here are some things to keep in mind:

Severity of Symptoms

The severity of a person's arthritis symptoms is often the most important factor in determining whether surgery is necessary. If someone is experiencing significant pain, stiffness, and loss of mobility that is impacting their daily life, surgery may be a viable option.

Non-surgical Treatments Have Not Worked

Before surgery is considered, it's important to exhaust all non-surgical treatment options first. This may include medication, physical therapy, bracing, and lifestyle modifications. If these treatments have not provided adequate relief, surgery may be necessary.

Joint Damage

Surgery may also be necessary if there is significant joint damage that cannot be repaired with non-surgical treatments. In some cases, joint replacement surgery may be the best option to improve joint function and alleviate pain.

Age and Overall Health

Age and overall health can also be important factors to consider when deciding whether to undergo surgery. Older adults may have a higher risk of complications during surgery, and those with pre-existing medical conditions may need to be evaluated carefully before undergoing any surgical procedures.

Types of Surgery for Arthritis

There are several different types of surgeries that may be considered for arthritis, depending on the severity of the condition and the specific joint affected. Here are a few examples:

Arthroscopy

Arthroscopy is a minimally invasive surgical procedure that involves inserting a small camera into the joint to assess the extent of the damage. This procedure may be used to remove damaged tissue or bone spurs that are causing pain and inflammation.

Joint Fusion

Joint fusion is a procedure in which the bones in a joint are fused together to eliminate motion and reduce pain. This may be an option for people with severe arthritis who have not found relief with other treatments.

Joint Replacement

Joint replacement surgery involves removing damaged bone and cartilage in the affected joint and replacing it with an artificial joint made of metal and plastic. This is often used for hips and knees, but may also be used for other joints such as the shoulder or elbow.

Osteotomy

Osteotomy involves cutting and reshaping the bone to shift weight-bearing away from the damaged portion of the joint. This may be an option for people with mild to moderate arthritis who are not yet candidates for joint replacement surgery.

Benefits and Risks of Surgery for Arthritis

While surgery can be an effective way to relieve arthritis symptoms and improve joint function, it is not without risks. Here are some potential benefits and risks of arthritis surgery:

Benefits:

Reduced pain and stiffness

Improved joint function and mobility

Increased quality of life

Reduced need for medication

Risks:

Infection

Blood clots

Nerve damage

Implant failure

Longer recovery time

It's important for people considering surgery for arthritis to discuss the potential benefits and risks with their healthcare provider and make an informed decision based on their individual needs and circumstances.

Types of joint replacement surgeries

Joint replacement surgery is a common treatment for advanced arthritis that cannot be effectively managed through other methods. There are several types of joint replacement surgeries that can be performed, depending on the type of arthritis and the affected joint.

Hip Replacement Surgery:

Hip replacement surgery involves replacing the hip joint with a prosthetic joint made of metal, plastic, or ceramic. This surgery is most commonly used to treat osteoarthritis, but it can also be used to treat other types of arthritis, such as rheumatoid arthritis. Hip replacement surgery can improve mobility, relieve pain, and improve quality of life for many patients.

Knee Replacement Surgery:

Knee replacement surgery involves replacing the knee joint with a prosthetic joint made of metal, plastic, or ceramic. This surgery is most commonly used to treat osteoarthritis, but it can also be used to treat other types of arthritis, such as rheumatoid arthritis. Knee replacement surgery can improve mobility, relieve pain, and improve quality of life for many patients.

Shoulder Replacement Surgery:

Shoulder replacement surgery involves replacing the shoulder joint with a prosthetic joint made of metal, plastic, or ceramic. This surgery is most commonly used to treat osteoarthritis, but it can also be used to treat other types of arthritis, such as rheumatoid arthritis. Shoulder replacement surgery can improve mobility, relieve pain, and improve quality of life for many patients.

Hand and Wrist Replacement Surgery:

Hand and wrist replacement surgery involves replacing the affected joint with a prosthetic joint made of metal, plastic, or ceramic. This surgery is most commonly used to treat rheumatoid arthritis, but it can also be used to treat other types of arthritis, such as osteoarthritis. Hand and wrist replacement surgery can improve mobility, relieve pain, and improve quality of life for many patients.

Ankle Replacement Surgery:

Ankle replacement surgery involves replacing the ankle joint with a prosthetic joint made of metal, plastic, or ceramic. This surgery is most commonly used to treat osteoarthritis, but it can also be used to treat other types of arthritis, such as rheumatoid arthritis. Ankle replacement surgery can improve mobility, relieve pain, and improve quality of life for many patients.

Spine Surgery:

Spine surgery is a less common type of joint replacement surgery that is used to treat severe cases of arthritis in the spine. This surgery involves replacing one or more vertebrae with a prosthetic joint made of metal or plastic. Spine surgery can improve mobility, relieve pain, and improve quality of life for many patients.

Joint replacement surgery can be a highly effective treatment for advanced arthritis, but it is not appropriate for everyone. Patients who are considering joint replacement surgery should work closely with their healthcare team to determine if this type of surgery is appropriate for them and what type of surgery would be best for their individual needs. It is important for patients to have realistic expectations for the outcome of the surgery and to understand the risks and potential complications associated with joint replacement surgery.

Recovery and rehabilitation

Arthritis is a common condition that can cause pain, stiffness, and swelling in the joints. In some cases, the condition can become severe enough that it interferes with daily activities, and surgery may be necessary. Joint replacement surgery is a common treatment for severe arthritis that can improve mobility and reduce pain. However, it is important to understand that joint replacement surgery is a major operation that requires careful planning and rehabilitation.

After joint replacement surgery, patients will spend some time in the hospital recovering from the surgery itself. Pain management is a critical component of this early recovery period, and medications will be prescribed to manage pain and swelling. Patients may be encouraged to begin moving their new joint as soon as possible to promote healing and prevent stiffness. Physical therapy may also be recommended to help with range of motion exercises and build strength in the affected area.

As patients begin to recover, they will work closely with their healthcare team to develop a rehabilitation plan that is tailored to their individual needs. Rehabilitation will typically involve a combination of exercises and therapies designed to help the patient regain strength and mobility in the affected joint. Patients may also work with an occupational therapist to learn techniques for performing everyday activities while protecting their new joint.

The recovery process can be lengthy, and it is important for patients to be patient and committed to their rehabilitation plan. Physical therapy sessions may be scheduled several times a week, and patients may need to continue exercising at home between appointments. It is important to follow all instructions from the healthcare team, including any restrictions on activity, to ensure the best possible outcome.

In addition to physical therapy and exercise, patients may also be advised to make certain lifestyle changes to support their recovery. For example, smoking can interfere with the healing process and increase the risk of complications, so patients may be encouraged to quit smoking prior to surgery. Additionally, maintaining a healthy weight can reduce stress on the joints and improve overall health.

It is important for patients to be aware of potential complications associated with joint replacement surgery, including infection, blood clots, and joint dislocation. Patients should be vigilant about any signs of infection, such as redness, swelling, or warmth around the incision site, and contact their healthcare provider if they suspect a problem. Patients should also take steps to reduce the risk of blood clots, such as wearing compression stockings and taking blood thinning medications as prescribed.

Chapter Sixteen

Prevention and Early Intervention

Prevention and early intervention are crucial when it comes to managing arthritis. Arthritis is a chronic disease that affects the joints, causing pain, stiffness, and decreased mobility. It can be caused by a variety of factors, including genetics, age, and injury. While there is no cure for arthritis, there are several ways to prevent or delay its onset and manage its symptoms.

The first step in preventing arthritis is maintaining a healthy lifestyle. Eating a balanced diet, getting regular exercise, and avoiding smoking and excessive alcohol consumption can help reduce the risk of developing arthritis. Maintaining a healthy weight is also important, as excess weight puts added pressure on the joints, increasing the risk of developing arthritis.

Regular exercise is important not only for maintaining a healthy weight but also for preventing arthritis. Exercise helps to strengthen the muscles and joints, improving flexibility and reducing the risk of injury. Low-impact exercises such as swimming, walking, and yoga are especially helpful for preventing arthritis.

In addition to maintaining a healthy lifestyle, early intervention is important when it comes to managing arthritis. If you experience joint pain or stiffness, it is important to see a doctor as soon as possible. Early intervention can help prevent further joint damage and reduce the risk of developing complications such as joint deformities.

There are several treatments available for arthritis, including medication, physical therapy, and surgery. Medications such as nonsteroidal anti-inflammatory drugs (NSAIDs) and disease-modifying antirheumatic drugs (DMARDs) can help manage pain and inflammation. Physical therapy can help improve flexibility and range of motion, while surgery can be used to repair or replace damaged joints.

In addition to these treatments, there are several other steps you can take to manage arthritis symptoms. Using assistive devices such as braces, splints, or canes can help reduce pressure on the joints, reducing pain and stiffness. Making modifications to your home or workplace, such as installing handrails or using ergonomic chairs, can also help reduce joint stress.

Stress management techniques such as meditation or deep breathing exercises can also be helpful for managing arthritis symptoms. Stress can exacerbate arthritis symptoms, so finding ways to manage stress can be beneficial.

Identifying risk factors

Arthritis is a common condition affecting millions of people worldwide. It is a leading cause of disability and can significantly affect one's quality of life. Although arthritis can develop at any age, it is more commonly seen in older adults. While there are various treatments available for arthritis, preventing or reducing the risk of developing it is the most effective way to manage the condition. One of the key steps in preventing arthritis is identifying the risk factors associated with the condition.

There are various risk factors that can contribute to the development of arthritis. These include genetics, age, gender, obesity, previous joint injury, and certain infections. People with a family history of arthritis are at a higher risk of developing the condition. Similarly, the likelihood of developing arthritis increases with age, with the majority of cases being seen in people over the age of 65. Women are also more likely to develop arthritis than men, particularly in the case of certain types of arthritis such as rheumatoid arthritis.

Obesity is another significant risk factor for developing arthritis. Excess weight places added stress on the joints, particularly in the knees and hips, increasing the risk of developing arthritis in those joints. Injuries to joints, particularly those that were not appropriately treated, can also lead to the development of arthritis in later life. Finally, certain infections, particularly those affecting the joints, can increase the risk of developing arthritis.

Identifying these risk factors is essential in developing prevention strategies for arthritis. People with a family history of arthritis should be aware of their increased risk and take appropriate measures to reduce their risk. This may include maintaining a healthy weight, staying active, and seeking medical advice if symptoms develop. Similarly, older adults and women should be aware of their increased risk and take appropriate measures to prevent the development of arthritis. This may include regular exercise, maintaining a healthy weight, and regular medical check-ups.

For those who have already developed arthritis or are at risk of developing the condition, early intervention is key. This involves identifying the symptoms of arthritis and seeking appropriate medical advice as soon as possible. Early diagnosis and treatment can help slow the progression of the disease and reduce the risk of complications.

Some of the common symptoms of arthritis include joint pain, stiffness, swelling, and reduced range of motion. These symptoms may be mild initially, but they tend to worsen over time. It is essential to seek medical advice if these symptoms persist for more than a few weeks, particularly if there is a family history of arthritis or other risk factors are present.

Once diagnosed, treatment for arthritis may involve a combination of lifestyle changes, medication, and physical therapy. Maintaining a healthy weight, regular exercise, and a healthy diet can help reduce the symptoms of arthritis and slow the progression of the disease. Medications such as nonsteroidal anti-inflammatory drugs (NSAIDs), disease-modifying antirheumatic drugs (DMARDs), and biologic agents may be prescribed to manage the symptoms of arthritis. Physical therapy, including exercises to improve strength and flexibility, may also be recommended.

Strategies for reducing arthritis risk

Arthritis is a common condition that affects millions of people worldwide. While it can be challenging to manage, there are strategies that can help to reduce the risk of developing arthritis or manage its symptoms. Below we will discuss some of the strategies for reducing arthritis risk.

Maintaining a healthy weight is one of the most important things you can do to reduce your risk of arthritis. Being overweight or obese puts extra stress on your joints, particularly the weight-bearing joints such as the hips, knees, and ankles. This stress can lead to wear and tear on the joints, which can contribute to the development of arthritis. By maintaining a healthy weight through a balanced diet and regular exercise, you can help to reduce this risk.

Exercise is also an essential component of arthritis prevention. Regular physical activity can help to keep your joints flexible and reduce stiffness. It can also help to build up the muscles that support your joints, which can help to protect them from damage. Exercises that are particularly helpful for reducing arthritis risk include low-impact activities such as walking, swimming, and cycling.

Another way to reduce arthritis risk is to practice good posture and ergonomics. Poor posture can put undue stress on your joints, particularly those in your neck, back, and hips. By practicing good posture, you can help to reduce this stress and prevent joint damage. Similarly, using ergonomic equipment, such as a supportive chair or computer mouse, can help to reduce the strain on your joints.

In addition to these strategies, it's also important to be aware of your joint health and to seek early intervention if you notice any signs of joint pain or stiffness. Arthritis can be a progressive condition, and early intervention can help to slow or even stop its progression. By seeing your doctor or a rheumatologist at the first sign of joint pain or stiffness, you can receive prompt treatment and improve your chances of preventing or managing arthritis.

Some early intervention strategies for managing arthritis symptoms include physical therapy, medications, and lifestyle modifications. Physical therapy can help to reduce joint stiffness and pain by improving joint flexibility and strength. Medications, such as nonsteroidal anti-inflammatory drugs (NSAIDs), can help to reduce inflammation and pain. Lifestyle modifications, such as dietary changes or stress reduction techniques, can also help to manage arthritis symptoms and improve overall joint health.

The importance of early intervention

Arthritis is a chronic condition that affects the joints and can cause pain, stiffness, and swelling. While there are many different types of arthritis, most forms develop slowly over time and become more common with age. Despite the fact that arthritis is a progressive condition, there are steps that can be taken to reduce the risk of developing arthritis or slow its progression, and one of the most important is early intervention.

The importance of early intervention in arthritis cannot be overstated. The earlier the condition is diagnosed and treated, the better the chances of slowing its progression and preventing or delaying long-term damage to the joints. In fact, the goal of early intervention is to achieve remission or low disease activity, which can significantly improve a patient's quality of life and reduce the risk of disability.

So, what steps can be taken to achieve early intervention in arthritis? One of the most important is to be aware of the risk factors for arthritis and to take steps to reduce them. These risk factors include age, family history, gender, obesity, joint injuries, and certain occupations that involve repetitive motions or heavy lifting. While some risk factors cannot be controlled, such as age and family history, there are steps that can be taken to reduce the risk of developing arthritis or slow its progression.

One of the most important steps is to maintain a healthy weight. Obesity is a major risk factor for arthritis, particularly in the knees and hips, as excess weight places additional stress on these joints. By maintaining a healthy weight through diet and exercise, individuals can reduce their risk of developing arthritis or slow its progression if it has already developed.

Another important step is to engage in regular physical activity. Exercise can help to strengthen the muscles around the joints, improve flexibility and range of motion, and reduce pain and stiffness. It is important to choose low-impact exercises, such as swimming, walking, or cycling, to reduce the risk of injury to the joints.

In addition to maintaining a healthy weight and engaging in regular physical activity, it is also important to protect the joints from injury. This can be achieved by avoiding repetitive motions that can cause joint damage, such as lifting heavy objects, and using proper ergonomics in the workplace.

Finally, it is important to seek medical attention as soon as symptoms of arthritis appear. This may include pain, stiffness, swelling, or decreased range of motion in the joints. Early diagnosis and treatment can significantly improve outcomes and prevent long-term damage to the joints.

The treatment options for arthritis depend on the type and severity of the condition. In some cases, lifestyle modifications such as weight loss, exercise, and joint protection may be enough to slow the progression of the condition and reduce symptoms. In more severe cases, medication or surgery may be necessary.

Medications commonly used to treat arthritis include nonsteroidal anti-inflammatory drugs (NSAIDs), disease-modifying antirheumatic drugs (DMARDs), and biologic agents. These medications can help to reduce inflammation, relieve pain, and slow the progression of the disease.

Surgery may be necessary in cases where the joints are severely damaged and conservative treatments are no longer effective. Joint replacement surgery, such as hip or knee replacement, can be an effective treatment for severe arthritis and can significantly improve quality of life.

Chapter Seventeen

Research and Future Therapies

Arthritis is a common condition that affects millions of people worldwide, causing pain, stiffness, and inflammation in the joints. While there are many treatments available, including medication, exercise, and surgery, researchers are always looking for new and innovative therapies to help those with arthritis manage their symptoms and improve their quality of life. Below we will explore some of the latest research in the field of arthritis and the potential future therapies that could change the way this condition is managed.

One area of research that has shown promise in the treatment of arthritis is the use of stem cells. Stem cells are special cells in the body that can differentiate into different types of cells, and researchers believe that they may hold the key to regenerating damaged cartilage and joint tissue. In recent studies, stem cell therapy has been used to successfully treat osteoarthritis, with patients experiencing less pain and increased joint function. While more research is needed to fully understand the potential of stem cell therapy, it could one day become a standard treatment for arthritis.

Another area of research that is gaining attention in the field of arthritis is the use of gene therapy. Gene therapy involves altering a patient's genes to treat or prevent disease, and researchers believe that it could be used to target the specific genes that contribute to the development of arthritis. By blocking or altering these genes, it may be possible to slow or even prevent the progression of the disease. While gene therapy is still in the experimental stages, it holds great potential for the future of arthritis treatment.

In addition to these cutting-edge therapies, there are also several other potential treatments that are currently being studied. For example, researchers are exploring the use of nanotechnology to deliver medications directly to the affected joints, which could help to reduce side effects and improve efficacy. There is also ongoing research into the role of the microbiome in arthritis, with some scientists believing that a better understanding of the bacteria and other microorganisms that live in the gut could lead to new treatment options.

While these future therapies hold great promise, it is important to remember that they are still in the experimental stages and may not be widely available for many years. In the meantime, there are several existing treatments that have been shown to be effective in managing arthritis symptoms. These include medication, physical therapy, and lifestyle changes such as diet and exercise.

One area of current research that is focused on improving these existing treatments is the use of personalized medicine. Personalized medicine involves tailoring treatments to individual patients based on their unique characteristics, such as their genetics, lifestyle, and medical history. By taking a more personalized approach to arthritis treatment, doctors may be able to improve outcomes and reduce side effects.

In addition to these treatment options, there is also ongoing research into the prevention of arthritis. As with many health conditions, early intervention is key to preventing the onset and progression of arthritis. Researchers are studying ways to identify those at risk for developing the condition, as well as strategies to reduce the risk of developing arthritis in the first place.

Current arthritis research

Arthritis is a complex condition that affects millions of people worldwide. With over 100 different types of arthritis, researchers have spent years working to better understand the causes, symptoms, and treatments of this condition. Current arthritis research is focusing on a variety of different areas, including genetics, inflammation, and new treatment options.

One area of arthritis research that has seen significant progress in recent years is genetics. Researchers have identified several genes that appear to increase the risk of developing certain types of arthritis. For example, a gene called HLA-B27 is strongly associated with ankylosing spondylitis, a type of arthritis that primarily affects the spine. Another gene called the shared epitope is associated with an increased risk of developing rheumatoid arthritis. These genetic findings are helping researchers to better understand the underlying causes of arthritis and to develop new therapies that target specific genetic pathways.

Another area of arthritis research that has seen significant progress in recent years is inflammation. Inflammation is a key component of arthritis, and researchers are working to better understand the underlying mechanisms of inflammation in the joints. This research has led to the development of new drugs called biologics that specifically target the inflammatory pathways involved in arthritis. Biologics have been shown to be effective in reducing inflammation and improving symptoms in many patients with rheumatoid arthritis, psoriatic arthritis, and other forms of inflammatory arthritis.

Researchers are also exploring new treatment options for arthritis, including stem cell therapy and gene therapy. Stem cell therapy involves using stem cells to regenerate damaged tissue in the joints. Early studies have shown promising results for stem cell therapy in the treatment of osteoarthritis, but more research is needed to fully understand its potential benefits and risks. Gene therapy involves using genetic engineering to modify cells in the body to produce therapeutic proteins that can reduce inflammation and promote tissue regeneration. While gene therapy is still in the early stages of development, it has the potential to be a powerful new treatment option for arthritis and other inflammatory conditions.

In addition to these areas of research, there are also ongoing studies exploring the role of diet, exercise, and other lifestyle factors in the prevention and treatment of arthritis. For example, some studies have suggested that certain foods, such as fatty fish and fruits and vegetables, may help to reduce inflammation in the body and improve arthritis symptoms. Other studies have explored the benefits of exercise and physical therapy for improving joint function and reducing pain in arthritis patients.

As researchers continue to explore these different areas of arthritis research, the hope is that new treatments and therapies will emerge that can improve the lives of millions of people living with arthritis. While there is still much to be learned about this complex condition, the progress being made in arthritis research is truly remarkable. By working together, researchers, healthcare providers, and patients can continue to advance our understanding of arthritis and develop new treatments that can help to reduce pain, improve function, and enhance overall quality of life.

Potential future treatments

Arthritis is a complex condition that affects millions of people worldwide. While there are several treatments available for arthritis, there is still a need for more effective and targeted therapies. This is where ongoing research comes in. Scientists and researchers are continually studying arthritis to better understand its causes and develop new treatments. Below we will discuss some of the potential future treatments for arthritis that are currently being researched.

One promising area of research is biologics. Biologics are a type of medication that targets specific components of the immune system that are responsible for inflammation. These medications are usually given by injection and can help reduce the symptoms of arthritis by targeting the underlying causes of inflammation. Biologics have been shown to be effective in treating several types of arthritis, including rheumatoid arthritis and psoriatic arthritis. However, they can be expensive and may have side effects, including an increased risk of infections.

Another area of research is stem cell therapy. Stem cells are cells that can develop into different types of cells in the body. Stem cell therapy involves injecting stem cells into the affected joint to help repair damaged tissue and reduce inflammation. This treatment is still in the early stages of research, but it shows promise in treating osteoarthritis and other types of arthritis.

Gene therapy is another area of research that could potentially lead to new treatments for arthritis. Gene therapy involves altering the genes responsible for the inflammation that causes arthritis. This could involve either silencing the genes responsible for inflammation or replacing them with genes that suppress inflammation. While gene therapy is still in the early stages of research, it could potentially lead to a more targeted and effective treatment for arthritis.

Researchers are also exploring the use of nanoparticles to deliver medications directly to the affected joint. Nanoparticles are tiny particles that can be engineered to carry medications and other therapeutic agents directly to the site of inflammation. This approach could potentially reduce the side effects of medications by targeting them specifically to the affected joint.

Nanoparticles are still being studied, but they have shown promise in early research.

In addition to these specific treatments, researchers are also exploring ways to improve current therapies for arthritis. For example, researchers are working to develop more effective pain medications that have fewer side effects than current medications. They are also exploring ways to improve joint replacement surgeries to make them more effective and less invasive.

While there is still much research to be done, these potential future treatments offer hope for people living with arthritis. By better understanding the causes of arthritis and developing new, targeted treatments, researchers hope to improve the lives of millions of people around the world.

The role of technology in arthritis management

The role of technology in arthritis management is becoming increasingly important as new advancements are being made to improve the lives of those living with arthritis. Arthritis is a chronic condition that affects millions of people worldwide and can lead to pain, stiffness, and swelling in the joints. While there is currently no cure for arthritis, technological innovations are helping individuals manage their symptoms and improve their overall quality of life.

One of the most significant advances in arthritis management technology is the development of wearable devices. Wearable devices are small, electronic devices that are worn on the body and can collect data on a person's physical activity, sleep, and other vital signs. For people with arthritis, wearable devices can be especially useful as they can help monitor joint movements and provide feedback on range of motion, which can be essential in managing symptoms.

Another important development in arthritis technology is the use of mobile apps. Many mobile apps have been developed to help individuals track their symptoms, set goals, and monitor their progress. Some of these apps even allow users to connect with healthcare professionals, share their data, and receive personalized recommendations for managing their symptoms. The use of mobile apps has proven to be an effective tool in helping individuals manage their arthritis symptoms and improve their overall quality of life.

Telemedicine is another technological advancement that has been increasingly used in arthritis management. Telemedicine refers to the use of telecommunications technology, such as video conferencing, to provide healthcare services remotely. For individuals with arthritis who may have mobility issues or live in remote areas, telemedicine can be a valuable tool in receiving regular medical care and staying connected with healthcare professionals.

Advancements in medical imaging technology have also been instrumental in arthritis management. X-rays, magnetic resonance imaging (MRI), and computed tomography (CT) scans are some of the imaging technologies used to diagnose and monitor arthritis. These imaging technologies can provide detailed images of joints, bones, and soft tissues, which can help healthcare professionals identify changes and monitor disease progression. The use of medical imaging has become increasingly important in the early diagnosis and treatment of arthritis.

Finally, robotics and exoskeletons have shown promising results in arthritis management. Robotic devices can help individuals with arthritis perform repetitive tasks, such as brushing teeth or opening jars, and reduce the strain on their joints. Exoskeletons are wearable devices that can provide support to joints and muscles, which can help reduce pain and increase mobility. Both robotics and exoskeletons have the potential to improve the quality of life for individuals with arthritis by increasing their independence and reducing pain and discomfort.

Chapter Eighteen

Travel and Leisure

Arthritis can be a challenging condition that affects people of all ages, but that doesn't mean that it has to put a stop to your travel and leisure plans. With some careful planning and preparation, it is possible to enjoy a variety of activities and destinations while managing arthritis symptoms. Below we will explore some tips and strategies for traveling and engaging in leisure activities with arthritis.

One of the first steps to successfully managing arthritis while traveling or engaging in leisure activities is to understand your limitations and plan accordingly. It may be helpful to consult with your healthcare provider prior to travel to discuss any concerns or limitations that you may have. They may be able to provide advice on activities or destinations that may be more suitable for your condition.

When planning your travel or leisure activities, consider the mode of transportation and accommodations. If you are traveling by plane or train, be sure to request any accommodations that may make your trip more comfortable, such as extra legroom or a special seat cushion. Additionally, if you will be staying in a hotel or other accommodations, be sure to request a room that is accessible and meets your needs. This may include a room with a bathtub instead of a shower or a room on the first floor if you have difficulty with stairs.

When it comes to engaging in leisure activities, it is important to choose activities that are suitable for your level of mobility and fitness. For example, hiking may be too strenuous for someone with advanced arthritis, but swimming or gentle yoga may be a more suitable option. Many tourist destinations offer activities that are tailored to those with disabilities or limited mobility, such as accessible hiking trails or adaptive equipment for water sports.

It is also important to pace yourself and take breaks as needed. If you are engaging in an activity that requires standing or walking for extended periods of time, be sure to take frequent breaks to rest and stretch. If you are traveling to a destination that requires a lot of walking, consider renting a mobility aid such as a wheelchair or scooter to help conserve your energy.

In addition to planning ahead for travel and leisure activities, there are also steps that can be taken to manage arthritis symptoms while on the go. One of the most important strategies is to continue with your regular exercise routine. This may include stretching or gentle exercise in the morning or evening, or finding a local gym or fitness center that offers equipment or classes suitable for those with arthritis.

It may also be helpful to pack any medications or supplements that you need to manage your arthritis symptoms, along with any assistive devices or equipment that you rely on at home. This may include items such as heating pads or ice packs, orthotics or braces, or a special cushion or pillow to help with comfort and support.

Finally, it is important to be prepared for unexpected changes or challenges while traveling or engaging in leisure activities. This may include unexpected weather changes or flight delays, or the need to adjust plans due to increased arthritis symptoms. It may be helpful to have a backup plan or alternative activities in mind in case of unexpected changes, and to remain flexible and adaptable in the face of challenges.

Planning for travel

Planning for Travel with Arthritis

Arthritis is a chronic condition that can cause pain, stiffness, and swelling in joints. It can affect people of all ages, including those who love to travel. For people with arthritis, traveling can be challenging, but it doesn't have to be impossible. With careful planning and preparation, people with arthritis can enjoy travel while managing their symptoms.

Below we will discuss the importance of planning for travel with arthritis and provide tips on how to make travel more comfortable and enjoyable.

The Importance of Planning

Before embarking on any trip, it's essential to plan ahead, especially for people with arthritis. Planning can help identify potential challenges and prevent potential problems. Here are some things to consider when planning for travel with arthritis:

1. Destination: Consider the destination's climate, terrain, and availability of medical facilities.

2. Mode of transportation: Choose a mode of transportation that will provide comfort and accommodate special needs.

3. Accommodations: Research and select accommodations that have easy access to the activities and attractions planned for the trip.

4. Medications: Make sure to pack all medications and any necessary medical supplies, including a copy of the prescription, in case they need to be refilled.

5. Packing: Pack light and only bring essential items. Use packing aids like compression bags or luggage with wheels to minimize stress on joints.

Tips for Traveling with Arthritis

Here are some tips to help make traveling with arthritis more comfortable and enjoyable:

6. Plan for breaks: When traveling long distances, plan for frequent breaks to stretch and move around. This can help alleviate stiffness and prevent pain.

7. Request accommodations: Contact airlines, hotels, and other travel providers ahead of time to request accommodations, such as a seat with extra legroom or a room on the ground floor.

8. Use assistive devices: Consider using assistive devices such as a cane, walker, or wheelchair to alleviate stress on joints.

9. Pack medications: Make sure to pack all medications and medical supplies in a carry-on bag to ensure they are easily accessible during travel.

10. Practice good posture: Maintain good posture during travel to reduce strain on joints. Sit up straight with shoulders back and feet flat on the floor.

11. Stay active: Keep moving and stretch regularly during travel to prevent stiffness and improve circulation.

12. Use heat or cold therapy: Bring a heat or cold pack to use during travel to alleviate pain and stiffness.

13. Avoid heavy lifting: When possible, avoid lifting heavy luggage or items that can cause strain on joints.

Tips for managing arthritis on vacation

Arthritis is a condition that causes inflammation in one or more joints. It can be a painful and debilitating condition that affects people of all ages, including those who are planning a vacation. Traveling with arthritis can be challenging, but with proper planning and preparation, it is possible to manage the condition and enjoy a relaxing vacation.

Here are some tips for managing arthritis on vacation:

Plan ahead

Before your trip, research your destination and plan your itinerary accordingly. Look for activities and attractions that are arthritis-friendly, such as museums, art galleries, and botanical gardens. Consider staying in a hotel that has amenities like a pool or spa, which can help soothe sore joints.

Pack wisely

Pack light and bring only the essentials. Choose luggage that is lightweight and easy to carry, such as a backpack or rolling suitcase. Pack comfortable and supportive shoes, as well as any medications, braces, or other aids that you may need.

Stay active

Although it may be tempting to spend your vacation lounging by the pool, staying active is important for managing arthritis. Look for activities that are low-impact and won't put too much strain on your joints. Walking, swimming, and yoga are all good options. If you are traveling by plane, make sure to get up and stretch your legs periodically to prevent stiffness.

Stay hydrated

Drinking plenty of water is important for everyone, but it is especially important for people with arthritis. Dehydration can make joint pain and inflammation worse, so make sure to drink plenty of water throughout the day.

Practice self-care

Traveling can be stressful, which can exacerbate arthritis symptoms. Take time to practice self-care, such as getting a massage or taking a relaxing bath. You can also bring along aromatherapy oils or a heating pad to help ease joint pain.

Use mobility aids

If you have difficulty walking or standing for long periods of time, consider using a mobility aid such as a cane or walker. You can also request wheelchair assistance at the airport or other transportation hubs.

Be mindful of your diet

Eating a healthy and balanced diet is important for managing arthritis. Try to avoid foods that are high in sugar, salt, and saturated fat, which can contribute to inflammation. Instead, focus on eating plenty of fruits, vegetables, whole grains, and lean protein.

Be prepared for emergencies

Make sure to bring a list of your medications and any important medical information with you on your trip. You should also research medical facilities in the area you will be visiting, in case of an emergency.

Accessible destinations and activities

As someone with arthritis, it's important to take into consideration the accessibility of your travel destination and planned activities. Fortunately, there are many destinations and activities that are accommodating to people with arthritis.

One of the most important factors to consider when choosing a travel destination is the climate. Warm, dry climates can be beneficial for people with arthritis, as humidity and cold temperatures can exacerbate symptoms. Places like Arizona, southern California, and parts of Florida are popular destinations for those seeking relief from arthritis symptoms.

It's also important to consider the availability of accessible accommodations, such as hotels or vacation rentals with ground-floor or elevator access, wide doorways, and grab bars in the bathroom. Many hotel chains have also begun offering rooms with adjustable beds and other amenities specifically designed for people with disabilities.

When planning activities, it's important to choose ones that are low-impact and won't put excessive strain on the joints. Swimming and water aerobics can be a great way to exercise without putting pressure on the joints. Walking tours and light hiking can also be enjoyable and easy on the joints if done in moderation.

Many cities have attractions that are wheelchair accessible and have accommodations for those with disabilities. Museums, galleries, and other cultural institutions often have ramps and elevators for those who have difficulty with stairs. Some even offer free or discounted admission for people with disabilities.

It's also important to research the accessibility of transportation options at your destination. Many cities have public transportation systems that are wheelchair accessible, and ride-sharing services like Uber and Lyft often have options for riders with disabilities.

When traveling with arthritis, it's important to remember to pace yourself and take breaks when needed. It's also a good idea to bring along any assistive devices or medications that you may need. Planning ahead and choosing accessible destinations and activities can make for a more enjoyable and comfortable travel experience.

Chapter Nineteen

Financial and Insurance Considerations

Financial and insurance considerations are important for those with arthritis. This chronic condition can result in significant medical expenses and loss of income, which can cause financial strain on both individuals and families. Below we will explore the financial and insurance considerations that people with arthritis should keep in mind.

Firstly, it is important to understand the potential costs associated with managing arthritis. Arthritis treatment can include medications, physical therapy, assistive devices, and even surgery, all of which can add up quickly. The cost of these treatments can vary depending on the type of arthritis and the severity of the condition. For example, biologic medications, which are commonly used for rheumatoid arthritis, can cost thousands of dollars per month. It is important to discuss these costs with a healthcare provider and insurance company to understand what treatments are covered and what costs will need to be covered out of pocket.

Secondly, it is important to understand the types of insurance that can help with arthritis-related expenses. Health insurance is crucial for covering the costs of doctor visits, medications, and treatments. It is important to review insurance policies and understand what is covered, what is not covered, and what the out-of-pocket costs are. Medicare and Medicaid are two government-sponsored programs that may provide assistance for those with arthritis who meet certain eligibility criteria. Disability insurance can also be important for those who are unable to work due to their condition.

Thirdly, it is important to consider financial assistance programs that may be available. Many pharmaceutical companies offer patient assistance programs for those who cannot afford the cost of their medications. Non-profit organizations, such as the Arthritis Foundation, may also offer financial assistance for those with arthritis. It is important to research and understand what financial assistance programs are available and how to apply for them.

Fourthly, it is important to be proactive in managing finances and planning for the future. This may include creating a budget, saving for medical expenses, and considering long-term care insurance. It is also important to be aware of the potential impact of arthritis on employment and income. Some individuals with arthritis may need to make changes to their work schedule or career path, which can impact their income and financial stability.

Lastly, it is important to be aware of potential scams and fraud related to arthritis treatment and financial assistance programs. There have been cases of individuals and companies exploiting those with arthritis for financial gain. It is important to research and verify any companies or programs offering financial assistance or treatments for arthritis.

Navigating insurance coverage

Arthritis can be a challenging and costly condition to manage. As such, navigating insurance coverage is an essential part of ensuring that people with arthritis receive the care they need. Insurance can cover a range of arthritis-related services, including medication, physical therapy, joint replacement surgeries, and more. However, it can also be confusing to understand what is covered, what is not, and how to navigate the insurance system.

The first step in navigating insurance coverage for arthritis is to understand what type of insurance you have. There are various types of insurance, including private health insurance, Medicare, Medicaid, and others. Each insurance type has its own rules and regulations for coverage, and it is essential to understand what your insurance plan covers.

For people with private health insurance, coverage for arthritis-related care can vary widely depending on the plan. Some private insurance plans cover a range of arthritis treatments and services, including medications, physical therapy, and surgery. However, some plans may have limited coverage or high out-of-pocket costs, such as copays or deductibles. It is crucial to review the details of your insurance plan and speak with your insurance provider to understand what is covered and what is not.

Medicare is a federal health insurance program for people over 65 years of age or those with certain disabilities. Medicare coverage for arthritis-related care includes doctor visits, X-rays, physical therapy, and some medications. However, there may be limitations on coverage, such as the number of therapy sessions allowed or specific medications that are not covered. It is important to review your Medicare plan and speak with your healthcare provider to understand what is covered.

Medicaid is a joint federal and state program that provides health insurance to people with low incomes. Medicaid coverage for arthritis-related care varies by state, but it generally covers doctor visits, medications, and some therapies. However, there may be limitations on coverage or specific requirements for eligibility. It is important to review your state's Medicaid plan and speak with your healthcare provider to understand what is covered.

In addition to understanding your insurance plan, there are several strategies to help navigate insurance coverage for arthritis. These include:

1. Keep accurate records: Keep track of all healthcare expenses related to your arthritis, including doctor visits, medications, and therapies. This can help you determine what is covered by your insurance plan and identify any discrepancies in coverage.

2. Understand the appeals process: If your insurance provider denies coverage for a service or treatment, you have the right to appeal the decision. Understanding the appeals process and knowing your rights can help you advocate for the coverage you need.

3. Consider alternative coverage options: If you have limited insurance coverage for arthritis-related care, consider alternative coverage options, such as financial assistance programs or patient advocacy groups. These resources can help offset the cost of treatment and provide additional support.

4. Communicate with your healthcare provider: Your healthcare provider can be an essential resource in navigating insurance coverage for arthritis. They can provide guidance on what treatments and services are covered by your insurance plan and help you navigate the appeals process if needed.

5. Stay informed: Stay up to date on changes to your insurance plan and any new coverage options that may become available. This can help you make informed decisions about your arthritis-related care and ensure that you receive the coverage you need.

Managing medical expenses

1. Managing Medical Expenses: Tips for Individuals with Arthritis

Arthritis is a chronic condition that affects millions of people worldwide. It can cause pain, stiffness, and swelling in joints, making it difficult to perform everyday tasks. Managing arthritis can be a challenge, especially when it comes to medical expenses. The cost of arthritis treatment can be high, and it is essential to have a plan in place to manage these expenses effectively. Below we will discuss tips for managing medical expenses for individuals with arthritis.

Understand Your Insurance Coverage

The first step in managing medical expenses for arthritis is to understand your insurance coverage. Knowing what is covered and what is not covered can help you plan for medical expenses. Many insurance plans have different levels of coverage, such as deductible, copayments, and coinsurance. It is essential to understand these terms and how they apply to your policy.

Compare Treatment Options

When it comes to arthritis treatment, there are many options available, including medication, physical therapy, and surgery. However, the cost of these treatments can vary significantly. It is essential to discuss treatment options with your doctor and compare the costs of each option. Sometimes, a less expensive treatment option may be just as effective as a more expensive one.

Use Generic Medications

Many arthritis medications are available in generic form, which can be significantly less expensive than brand-name medications. Ask your doctor if there is a generic option for your medication and discuss the cost savings with your pharmacist.

Look for Financial Assistance Programs

Many pharmaceutical companies offer financial assistance programs to help individuals with the cost of their medications. These programs can provide free or reduced-cost medication to individuals who meet certain income and eligibility requirements. Additionally, some nonprofit organizations provide financial assistance to individuals with arthritis.

Take Advantage of Free Services

There are many free services available to individuals with arthritis that can help reduce medical expenses. For example, some hospitals and clinics offer free health screenings and medical consultations. Additionally, some organizations provide free or low-cost transportation services for individuals who have difficulty getting to medical appointments.

Use a Health Savings Account

A health savings account (HSA) is a tax-advantaged savings account that can be used to pay for medical expenses. HSAs are available to individuals who have a high-deductible health insurance plan. Money contributed to an HSA is tax-deductible, and withdrawals for qualified medical expenses are tax-free.

Consider Supplemental Insurance

Supplemental insurance, such as accident insurance or critical illness insurance, can provide additional coverage for medical expenses not covered by your primary insurance. These types of insurance policies can help pay for deductibles, copayments, and other out-of-pocket expenses associated with arthritis treatment.

Negotiate Medical Bills

If you receive a medical bill that is higher than you expected, don't be afraid to negotiate. Many healthcare providers are willing to work with patients to find a payment plan that fits their budget. Additionally, some hospitals and clinics offer financial assistance programs to individuals who meet certain income requirements.

Shop Around for Medical Services

The cost of medical services can vary significantly from one provider to another. Before scheduling a medical procedure, it is essential to shop around and compare prices. You may be able to find a provider that offers the same services at a lower cost.

Assistance programs and resources

Arthritis is a condition that affects millions of people worldwide, and managing its symptoms can be both physically and financially challenging. While there is no cure for arthritis, there are various treatments and resources available that can help those with the condition manage their symptoms and improve their quality of life. One of these resources is assistance programs and resources, which can help ease the financial burden of managing arthritis.

There are numerous assistance programs and resources available for people with arthritis. These programs can help with a variety of needs, from paying for medication to providing emotional support. Here are some of the most common programs and resources available:

1. Government programs: The government offers several programs that can provide financial assistance to people with arthritis. These programs include Medicaid, which provides health coverage to people with low incomes, and Medicare, which provides coverage for people over the age of 65 or those with certain disabilities. Additionally, the Social Security Disability Insurance program provides financial assistance to people who are unable to work due to a disability, including arthritis.

2. Non-profit organizations: There are many non-profit organizations that offer resources and support to people with arthritis. The Arthri-

tis Foundation is one such organization, offering educational materials, support groups, and advocacy initiatives. Other non-profit organizations, such as the National Psoriasis Foundation and the Lupus Foundation of America, offer resources and support to those with related conditions that often overlap with arthritis.

3. Pharmaceutical company programs: Many pharmaceutical companies offer patient assistance programs that provide financial assistance to those who cannot afford their medications. These programs often provide free or reduced-cost medications to eligible patients.

4. Charitable organizations: There are numerous charitable organizations that offer financial assistance to people with arthritis. For example, the Chronic Disease Fund provides financial assistance to people with chronic conditions, including arthritis, to help cover the cost of medications and other treatments.

5. Community resources: Local community resources can also be helpful for people with arthritis. For example, community centers often offer exercise classes specifically designed for people with arthritis, and local libraries may offer resources on managing arthritis symptoms.

In addition to these resources, there are several steps that people with arthritis can take to manage their medical expenses. Here are some tips:

6. Review insurance coverage: It is important to review insurance coverage to understand what is covered and what is not. Some insurance plans may cover certain treatments, such as physical therapy or acupuncture, that can help manage arthritis symptoms.

7. Consider generic medications: Generic medications are often less expensive than brand-name drugs and can be just as effective. Talk to a healthcare provider about whether generic medications are an option.

8. Shop around for the best prices: The cost of medications and treatments can vary widely between pharmacies and healthcare providers. Shopping around for the best prices can help save money.

9. Look for discounts and coupons: Many pharmacies and healthcare providers offer discounts and coupons that can help lower the cost of medications and treatments.

10. Take advantage of assistance programs and resources: As discussed above, there are numerous assistance programs and resources available to people with arthritis. Taking advantage of these programs can help ease the financial burden of managing arthritis.

Chapter Twenty

Overcoming Obstacles

Arthritis is a chronic condition that affects millions of people worldwide. It can cause a variety of physical and emotional challenges that can make daily life more difficult. However, it is possible to overcome these obstacles and live a fulfilling life with arthritis. Below we will explore some of the most common obstacles that people with arthritis face and offer strategies for overcoming them.

One of the biggest obstacles for people with arthritis is pain. Chronic pain can be debilitating, making it difficult to perform even basic tasks such as getting out of bed or taking a shower. While there is no cure for arthritis, there are several strategies that can help manage pain. For example, exercise can help alleviate pain and stiffness by strengthening the muscles around the affected joints. Low-impact exercises such as swimming or walking are great options for people with arthritis.

Another strategy for managing pain is to use hot or cold therapy. Applying a hot or cold pack to the affected joint can help reduce inflammation and alleviate pain. Physical therapy can also be helpful in managing pain, as it can help improve joint function and range of motion.

Fatigue is another common obstacle that people with arthritis face. Chronic fatigue can make it difficult to complete daily tasks or participate in social activities. To overcome this obstacle, it's important to pace oneself throughout the day and take breaks when needed. It may also be helpful to prioritize tasks and focus on the most important ones first.

Another strategy for managing fatigue is to practice good sleep hygiene. This includes establishing a regular sleep schedule, avoiding caffeine and alcohol before bed, and creating a relaxing sleep environment. Taking short naps throughout the day can also help alleviate fatigue.

Mobility issues can also be a challenge for people with arthritis. Joint pain and stiffness can make it difficult to walk or climb stairs. To overcome this obstacle, it may be necessary to make modifications to the home, such as installing handrails in the bathroom or adding a ramp to the front entrance. It may also be helpful to use assistive devices such as canes or walkers.

In addition, physical therapy can help improve mobility by strengthening the muscles around the affected joints. Exercises that focus on balance and coordination can also be helpful.

Depression and anxiety are common emotional challenges that people with arthritis face. The chronic pain and disability associated with arthritis can take a toll on one's mental health. To overcome these obstacles, it's important to seek support from loved ones and healthcare professionals. Joining a support group or talking to a mental health professional can also be helpful.

Exercise and physical activity can also help alleviate depression and anxiety by releasing endorphins and improving mood. Relaxation techniques such as deep breathing or meditation can also help reduce stress and anxiety.

Finally, financial concerns can be a major obstacle for people with arthritis. Medical bills and the cost of assistive devices and medication can add up quickly. It's important to explore all available resources, such as government assistance programs and insurance coverage.

Another strategy for managing medical expenses is to communicate with healthcare providers and ask about generic or less expensive medication options. It may also be helpful to explore alternative therapies such as acupuncture or massage therapy, which may be covered by insurance or offered at a reduced cost through community programs.

Resilience and adaptability

Resilience and adaptability are two key traits that can greatly benefit individuals living with arthritis. Arthritis can be a chronic condition, which means that it can be a long-term battle. It is important for individuals to understand that while there may be challenges, there are ways to manage and adapt to these challenges.

Resilience is the ability to bounce back from setbacks or challenges. It is the ability to face adversity with strength and perseverance. People with arthritis may face physical, emotional, and mental challenges. For instance, they may experience pain, fatigue, or limitations in mobility. Resilience helps individuals to manage these challenges with determination and courage.

Adaptability is the ability to adjust to new circumstances or situations. People with arthritis may need to adapt to changes in their body, in their lifestyle, and in their social activities. This may require changes in daily routines, activities, or relationships. Adaptability helps individuals to find new ways to approach tasks or challenges, and to find creative solutions to problems.

One way that people with arthritis can build resilience and adaptability is by adopting a positive mindset. This involves focusing on strengths rather than weaknesses, and looking for opportunities rather than limitations. It also means being patient with oneself and acknowledging that setbacks and mistakes are a normal part of life.

Another way to build resilience and adaptability is to develop a support network. This may include family, friends, healthcare professionals, or support groups. Having a support network can provide emotional and practical support, as well as advice and encouragement. It can also help individuals to stay motivated and focused on their goals.

Physical activity is another important factor in building resilience and adaptability. Exercise can help to improve physical strength, mobility, and flexibility. It can also boost mental health, reduce stress, and improve overall wellbeing. People with arthritis should talk to their healthcare provider about the types of exercises that are safe and effective for them.

Diet and nutrition also play a role in managing arthritis. Eating a healthy, balanced diet can provide the body with the nutrients it needs to support joint health and reduce inflammation. It is important to limit foods that are high in sugar, saturated fats, and processed foods. Foods that are rich in omega-3 fatty acids, such as fish, nuts, and seeds, can be beneficial for joint health.

In addition to these lifestyle factors, there are also medical treatments available for managing arthritis. These may include medications, physical therapy, and surgery. It is important for individuals to work closely with their healthcare provider to develop a treatment plan that is tailored to their individual needs and goals.

Finding motivation and purpose

Arthritis can be a challenging condition to live with, as it can cause chronic pain, stiffness, and fatigue. However, finding motivation and purpose can be a powerful tool in managing arthritis and improving overall well-being. Below we will explore various strategies for finding motivation and purpose while living with arthritis.

One of the key factors in finding motivation and purpose is setting achievable goals. When living with arthritis, it is important to set realistic goals that take into account the limitations of the condition. These goals can be related to physical activity, career, relationships, or hobbies, and can help to provide a sense of accomplishment and satisfaction.

Physical activity is an essential component of managing arthritis, as it can help to reduce pain and stiffness, improve flexibility, and enhance overall health. Setting goals related to physical activity can help to keep individuals motivated and engaged in their exercise routines. For example, a person with arthritis may set a goal to walk for 30 minutes each day, take a yoga class twice a week, or participate in a local charity walk.

Career goals can also provide a sense of purpose and motivation for individuals with arthritis. It is important to communicate with employers about the challenges of living with arthritis and to explore options for accommodations or flexible work arrangements. For example, a person with arthritis may work with their employer to establish a more ergonomic work station or to adjust their schedule to allow for rest breaks throughout the day.

Relationships can also provide a source of motivation and purpose. Spending time with loved ones, connecting with others who have similar experiences, and engaging in social activities can help to reduce feelings of isolation and loneliness that can sometimes accompany arthritis. Individuals with arthritis may find it helpful to join a support group or to participate in online forums where they can connect with others who understand what they are going through.

Hobbies and creative pursuits can also provide a sense of purpose and motivation. Engaging in activities that bring joy and fulfillment, such as painting, gardening, or playing music, can help to reduce stress and improve mood. It is important to find activities that are enjoyable and accessible, and to modify activities as necessary to accommodate physical limitations.

Another strategy for finding motivation and purpose is to focus on gratitude and positive thinking. Research has shown that practicing gratitude can improve well-being and resilience, even in the face of challenging circumstances. Taking time each day to reflect on what is going well, to express gratitude for the people and things in our lives, and to focus on positive aspects of our experiences can help to cultivate a sense of purpose and motivation.

In addition to these strategies, it is important to remember that seeking support when needed is a sign of strength, not weakness. Arthritis can be a challenging condition to manage, and it is important to reach out for help when necessary. This may involve working with a healthcare provider to explore treatment options, joining a support group or therapy program, or seeking assistance from family or friends.

Celebrating successes

Arthritis can be a challenging condition to live with, but it's important to remember that there are still opportunities for success and celebration. Success can mean different things to different people, but generally, it refers to achieving a desired goal or outcome. It's important for those with arthritis to celebrate their successes, no matter how big or small they may be. Below we will we'll discuss why celebrating successes is important, as well as some tips for how to do it.

Living with arthritis can be difficult and can make daily tasks seem like insurmountable challenges. This can lead to feelings of frustration, sadness, and a sense of hopelessness. Celebrating successes can help individuals with arthritis feel more positive and empowered. It can help them to see that they are capable of achieving their goals, despite the challenges they may face.

Celebrating successes can also be a way to acknowledge the hard work that has been put in to achieve a goal. Arthritis can make everyday tasks like cooking, cleaning, and even walking, feel like monumental feats. Celebrating the completion of these tasks, no matter how small they may seem, can be a way to recognize the effort that has been put in.

So, how can individuals with arthritis celebrate their successes? Here are some tips:

1. Keep a journal: Write down your successes, no matter how big or small. This can help you to see your progress and remind you of what you've achieved.

2. Share your successes with others: Share your successes with friends, family, or a support group. This can be a way to acknowledge your hard work and receive encouragement from others.

3. Treat yourself: Treat yourself to something special when you achieve a goal. This can be something as simple as a favorite snack or a day out doing something you love.

4. Focus on the positive: Try to focus on the positive aspects of your life and your accomplishments, rather than dwelling on what you haven't achieved.

5. Set achievable goals: Setting achievable goals can help to boost confidence and provide a sense of accomplishment. It's important to set goals that are realistic and attainable, even if they seem small.

6. Celebrate progress: Celebrate progress, not just the final outcome. It's important to recognize the effort that goes into achieving a goal, even if the final outcome isn't exactly what was expected.

7. Stay motivated: Use your successes as motivation to continue to work towards your goals. Remembering what you've achieved can help to keep you motivated and focused on what's important.

In addition to celebrating individual successes, it's also important to celebrate successes as a community. Organizations and individuals who work towards improving the lives of those with arthritis should be recognized and celebrated. This can include advocacy groups, researchers, and healthcare professionals who are dedicated to finding new treatments and therapies for arthritis.

Chapter Twenty-One

Arthritis and Mental Health

Arthritis is a chronic condition that affects millions of people worldwide. It can cause pain, swelling, and stiffness in the joints, which can lead to physical limitations and decreased quality of life. However, what many people don't realize is that arthritis can also have a significant impact on mental health.

The physical symptoms of arthritis can take a toll on a person's mental well-being. Chronic pain, fatigue, and mobility issues can lead to feelings of frustration, anxiety, and depression. The stress of managing a chronic illness can also lead to social isolation and decreased participation in activities that were once enjoyable.

Research has shown that individuals with arthritis are more likely to experience depression than those without the condition. One study found that up to 30% of people with arthritis also had symptoms of depression. Another study found that people with arthritis had a higher risk of anxiety disorders compared to those without arthritis.

The link between arthritis and mental health is complex, and the relationship is bidirectional. This means that arthritis can contribute to mental health issues, and mental health issues can also make arthritis symptoms worse. For example, depression can worsen pain perception, leading to increased physical discomfort.

Fortunately, there are strategies that individuals with arthritis can use to manage their mental health and improve their overall well-being. Here are some tips:

1. Seek support: Don't be afraid to talk to friends, family, or a mental health professional about your feelings. Joining a support group can also be helpful, as it can provide an opportunity to connect with others who are going through similar experiences.

2. Stay active: Physical activity has been shown to improve both physical and mental health. Low-impact exercises such as swimming, walking, or cycling can be beneficial for individuals with arthritis.

3. Practice relaxation techniques: Activities such as meditation, deep breathing, and yoga can help reduce stress and promote relaxation.

4. Engage in enjoyable activities: It's important to continue doing activities that bring joy and satisfaction. This can help combat feelings of social isolation and improve overall mood.

5. Address negative thoughts: It's common for individuals with arthritis to experience negative thoughts about their condition. However, these thoughts can worsen mental health. Cognitive-behavioral therapy (CBT) is a type of talk therapy that can help individuals identify and challenge negative thoughts.

6. Work with healthcare providers: Healthcare providers such as rheumatologists and mental health professionals can work together to create a treatment plan that addresses both physical and mental health needs.

In addition to these strategies, it's important to prioritize self-care and to seek help when needed. Arthritis can be a challenging condition to manage, but with the right support and resources, individuals can maintain their mental and physical health and live fulfilling lives.

The connection between arthritis and mental health

Arthritis is a chronic condition that affects millions of people around the world. It is a condition that can cause significant physical pain and limitations, as well as emotional stress and strain. The impact of arthritis on mental health is often overlooked or underestimated, but it can be just as significant as the physical symptoms.

The connection between arthritis and mental health is complex and multifaceted. Arthritis can cause pain, stiffness, and fatigue, which can make it difficult to perform daily activities. This can lead to feelings of frustration, helplessness, and even depression. Chronic pain is one of the most common symptoms of arthritis, and it can have a significant impact on mental health. It can lead to anxiety, depression, and other mood disorders.

Chronic pain can also make it difficult to sleep, which can exacerbate feelings of anxiety and depression. Lack of sleep can cause fatigue, irritability, and difficulty concentrating, which can further impact mental health. People with arthritis may also experience social isolation, as they may not be able to participate in activities that they once enjoyed. This can lead to feelings of loneliness and depression.

There are also several risk factors for mental health problems among people with arthritis. For example, people with arthritis are more likely to have other chronic health conditions, such as heart disease and diabetes, which can increase the risk of depression and anxiety. They may also be more likely to experience financial hardship, as arthritis can cause significant medical expenses and may impact their ability to work.

Fortunately, there are ways to manage the impact of arthritis on mental health. One of the most important steps is to seek support from family, friends, and healthcare professionals. Talking to someone about the challenges of living with arthritis can help to reduce feelings of isolation and frustration. It can also help to identify strategies for managing pain and fatigue.

There are also several evidence-based therapies that can be effective in treating mental health problems among people with arthritis. Cognitive-behavioral therapy (CBT) is a type of talk therapy that focuses on changing negative thought patterns and behaviors. It can be effective in reducing symptoms of depression and anxiety among people with arthritis.

Another effective therapy for people with arthritis is mindfulness-based stress reduction (MBSR). This is a type of meditation that involves focusing on the present moment and accepting one's thoughts and feelings without judgment. MBSR has been shown to be effective in reducing pain, anxiety, and depression among people with arthritis.

Exercise can also be an effective way to improve mental health among people with arthritis. Exercise has been shown to reduce symptoms of depression and anxiety, as well as improve sleep and reduce pain. People with arthritis may need to modify their exercise routine to accommodate their physical limitations, but there are many exercises that can be done safely and effectively.

In addition to seeking support and engaging in evidence-based therapies, there are several other strategies that can help to manage the impact of arthritis on mental health. These include:

1. Getting enough sleep: This can help to reduce fatigue and improve mood.

2. Eating a healthy diet: A healthy diet can help to reduce inflammation and improve overall health.

3. Engaging in relaxing activities: Activities such as yoga, meditation, and tai chi can help to reduce stress and promote relaxation.

4. Maintaining a positive attitude: It can be difficult to maintain a positive attitude when living with chronic pain and limitations, but focusing on the things that are still possible can help to improve mood and overall well-being.

Managing stress and anxiety

Arthritis can be a painful and challenging condition to manage, and it can often lead to stress and anxiety in individuals affected by it. Managing stress and anxiety is important in the overall management of arthritis as it can impact both physical and mental well-being. Below we will explore the connection between arthritis and mental health, and provide tips on managing stress and anxiety associated with arthritis.

Arthritis and Mental Health

Arthritis is a chronic condition that affects the joints and can cause pain, inflammation, stiffness, and loss of mobility. This condition can have a significant impact on a person's daily life, causing limitations in activities, decreased quality of life, and increased risk of depression and anxiety. Studies have found that individuals with arthritis are two to three times more likely to experience depression than those without arthritis. This connection between arthritis and mental health is complex and multifaceted.

One factor that contributes to the link between arthritis and mental health is the chronic pain associated with the condition. Arthritis pain can be debilitating, affecting the ability to carry out daily tasks and causing significant distress. This pain can lead to feelings of frustration, hopelessness, and helplessness, which can contribute to anxiety and depression.

Another factor is the impact of arthritis on daily activities and social functioning. Arthritis can limit mobility and make it difficult to participate in social activities, which can lead to feelings of isolation and loneliness. These feelings can further contribute to stress and anxiety.

Managing Stress and Anxiety

Managing stress and anxiety associated with arthritis is essential for overall well-being. Here are some tips that can help:

1. Exercise: Regular exercise can help reduce stress and anxiety, while also helping to improve joint mobility and overall physical health. Low-impact exercises like swimming, cycling, and walking can be particularly beneficial for individuals with arthritis.

2. Practice relaxation techniques: Techniques such as deep breathing, meditation, and yoga can help reduce stress and anxiety. These practices can also help improve sleep quality, which is essential for overall well-being.

3. Stay connected: Social support is important for managing stress and anxiety. Connecting with friends and family, joining support groups, and participating in community activities can help combat feelings of isolation and loneliness.

4. Get professional help: If stress and anxiety are interfering with daily life, it may be helpful to seek professional help. A mental health professional can provide strategies for managing stress and anxiety and help improve overall well-being.

5. Stay positive: Maintaining a positive outlook can help reduce stress and anxiety. Focus on the things that can be done, rather than dwelling on what cannot be changed. Celebrate small victories and successes.

Seeking professional help

Arthritis is a chronic condition that affects millions of people worldwide. It can cause pain, stiffness, and inflammation in the joints, making it difficult for individuals to perform daily activities. But arthritis doesn't just affect the physical body - it can also have a significant impact on mental health. Individuals with arthritis may experience feelings of anxiety, depression, and stress due to the constant pain and limitations that the condition brings. Below we will discuss the importance of seeking professional help for managing the mental health aspects of arthritis.

Arthritis can cause a great deal of emotional distress for those who suffer from it. The pain and stiffness can make it difficult to perform tasks that were once routine, leading to frustration and a feeling of loss of independence. Additionally, arthritis can make individuals feel isolated and alone, as they may not be able to participate in activities they once enjoyed with friends and family. These factors can lead to anxiety and depression, making it challenging to manage the physical symptoms of the condition.

It's important for individuals with arthritis to seek professional help for their mental health. This can include speaking with a therapist or counselor who can help individuals manage their emotions and develop coping strategies for dealing with the challenges of living with arthritis. Therapy can also provide a safe and supportive environment for individuals to express their fears and concerns about the condition and its impact on their lives.

Medication can also be used to manage the mental health aspects of arthritis. Antidepressants, anti-anxiety medications, and other medications used to manage mental health conditions can be effective in reducing symptoms of anxiety and depression in individuals with arthritis. However, it's essential to discuss any medication changes with a healthcare professional to ensure that they are safe and effective.

In addition to therapy and medication, lifestyle changes can also play a crucial role in managing mental health with arthritis. Exercise has been shown to have a positive impact on mental health, reducing stress and anxiety, and improving mood. Even gentle forms of exercise, such as walking or yoga, can be effective in managing mental health symptoms associated with arthritis.

Support groups can also be an essential resource for individuals with arthritis. These groups provide a sense of community and understanding for individuals who may feel alone or isolated in their experiences. Support groups can also offer practical advice and tips for managing the physical and mental aspects of arthritis.

Finally, it's important to recognize when professional help may be necessary. If feelings of anxiety or depression persist, despite attempts to manage them through therapy, medication, and lifestyle changes, it may be necessary to speak with a healthcare professional. They can help individuals explore additional treatment options, such as more intensive therapy or medication changes.

Chapter Twenty-Two

Sleep and Arthritis

Sleep and Arthritis

Arthritis is a common condition that affects millions of people worldwide. It can cause chronic pain and stiffness in joints, making it difficult to carry out daily activities. One of the most common complaints among people with arthritis is the inability to get a good night's sleep. Below we will explore the relationship between arthritis and sleep and provide tips on how to manage sleep disturbances related to arthritis.

The Connection between Arthritis and Sleep

Arthritis can interfere with sleep in several ways. Firstly, the pain and discomfort associated with arthritis can make it difficult to fall asleep or stay asleep throughout the night. People with arthritis may also wake up frequently during the night due to pain, stiffness, or other symptoms.

Secondly, certain medications used to manage arthritis symptoms can also disrupt sleep. For example, corticosteroids, a common medication used to reduce inflammation, can cause insomnia or other sleep disturbances.

Finally, arthritis can also cause mental health issues such as anxiety or depression, which can further impact sleep quality.

Sleep and Arthritis Management

Managing sleep disturbances related to arthritis can be challenging, but it is essential for overall well-being. The following are some tips for improving sleep quality:

Create a Sleep-Conducive Environment

Creating a comfortable sleeping environment is essential to ensure good sleep quality. This may include investing in a comfortable mattress and pillows, keeping the room at a comfortable temperature, and minimizing noise and light.

Stick to a Sleep Schedule

Establishing a regular sleep schedule can help regulate the body's internal clock and improve sleep quality. Going to bed and waking up at the same time each day can help improve sleep quality over time.

Incorporate Relaxation Techniques

Incorporating relaxation techniques such as deep breathing, meditation, or yoga can help reduce stress and promote relaxation, making it easier to fall asleep and stay asleep.

Exercise Regularly

Regular exercise can help manage arthritis symptoms and improve sleep quality. However, it is important to avoid exercising too close to bedtime, as it can stimulate the body and make it difficult to fall asleep.

Practice Good Sleep Hygiene

Practicing good sleep hygiene, such as avoiding caffeine and alcohol before bedtime, can help improve sleep quality. It is also important to avoid using electronic devices before bedtime, as the blue light emitted by these devices can interfere with the body's natural sleep-wake cycle.

Discuss Medications with a Healthcare Provider

If arthritis medications are interfering with sleep, it may be necessary to discuss alternative medications or adjust dosages with a healthcare provider. It is important to never stop taking medication without consulting a healthcare provider.

The importance of sleep for arthritis management

Arthritis is a condition that can cause chronic pain and stiffness in the joints, making it difficult for those affected to engage in regular activities, including getting enough sleep. While getting enough sleep is important for overall health, it is especially crucial for those with arthritis. Sleep helps to reduce inflammation, which is a key factor in arthritis pain, and it also allows the body to repair and regenerate damaged tissue.

Unfortunately, many people with arthritis struggle with sleep disturbances, including difficulty falling asleep, waking up frequently throughout the night, and waking up feeling tired and unrefreshed. This can create a vicious cycle of pain, as lack of sleep can increase inflammation and pain, making it even harder to sleep.

So, what can be done to improve sleep in people with arthritis? Here are some strategies to consider:

1. Develop a regular sleep routine: Going to bed and waking up at the same time every day can help to regulate the body's internal clock, making it easier to fall asleep and wake up feeling refreshed. Aim for 7-9 hours of sleep per night.

2. Create a comfortable sleep environment: Make sure your bedroom is dark, quiet, and cool, with comfortable bedding and pillows. Consider

using blackout curtains, earplugs, or a white noise machine to help block out distractions.

3. Practice relaxation techniques: Engage in relaxation techniques, such as deep breathing, meditation, or progressive muscle relaxation, to help calm the mind and body before bed.

4. Exercise regularly: Exercise can help to reduce arthritis pain and stiffness, and it can also improve sleep quality. Aim for at least 30 minutes of moderate exercise most days of the week, but avoid exercise close to bedtime as it can be stimulating.

5. Avoid caffeine and alcohol: Caffeine and alcohol can interfere with sleep, so avoid consuming them close to bedtime.

6. Use heat therapy: Heat therapy, such as taking a warm bath or using a heating pad on sore joints, can help to reduce pain and stiffness and promote relaxation.

7. Consider medication: If non-pharmacological strategies are not enough, talk to your doctor about medications that may help with sleep, such as sleep aids or low-dose antidepressants.

In addition to these strategies, it's important to address any underlying issues that may be contributing to poor sleep, such as stress or anxiety. Working with a healthcare provider or a mental health professional can help to identify and address these issues.

Tips for improving sleep quality

Arthritis is a condition that affects millions of people worldwide, and one of the most common symptoms of this condition is disrupted sleep. People with arthritis often struggle to fall asleep or stay asleep, which can negatively impact their overall health and well-being. However, there are several tips and strategies that people with arthritis can use to improve the quality of their sleep and reduce the impact of arthritis-related sleep disturbances.

The first step in improving sleep quality for people with arthritis is to create a comfortable sleep environment. This can include investing in a supportive mattress and pillow, using soft and breathable bedding, and ensuring that the bedroom is cool and quiet. It's also important to minimize distractions and sources of stress in the bedroom, such as televisions or computers.

In addition to creating a comfortable sleep environment, people with arthritis can benefit from establishing a consistent sleep routine. Going to bed and waking up at the same time each day can help regulate the body's internal clock and promote more restful sleep. It's also important to avoid napping during the day, as this can disrupt the body's natural sleep-wake cycle.

Another tip for improving sleep quality is to engage in relaxation techniques before bed. This can include deep breathing exercises, meditation, or gentle stretching. These activities can help reduce stress and tension in the body, making it easier to fall asleep and stay asleep throughout the night.

Physical activity during the day can also improve sleep quality for people with arthritis. Regular exercise can help reduce joint pain and stiffness, which can make it easier to fall asleep and stay asleep. However, it's important to avoid intense or strenuous exercise close to bedtime, as this can increase alertness and make it more difficult to fall asleep.

For people with arthritis, pain management is often a key component of improving sleep quality. Pain can interfere with sleep by making it difficult to find a comfortable sleeping position or causing frequent awakenings throughout the night. Over-the-counter pain relievers, such as acetaminophen or nonsteroidal anti-inflammatory drugs (NSAIDs), may be helpful for managing arthritis pain and improving sleep quality. However, it's important to consult with a healthcare provider before starting any new medication, as some medications can have side effects or interact with other medications.

Finally, cognitive-behavioral therapy (CBT) can be a helpful tool for managing sleep disturbances related to arthritis. CBT is a type of therapy that focuses on changing negative thought patterns and behaviors that may be contributing to sleep problems. A trained therapist can help people with arthritis identify and address underlying issues that may be interfering with sleep, such as anxiety, depression, or chronic pain.

Managing sleep disturbances

Arthritis is a condition that affects the joints, causing pain, stiffness, and limited mobility. It can make it difficult for people to carry out everyday activities, including getting enough restful sleep. Unfortunately, many people with arthritis experience sleep disturbances, which can exacerbate their symptoms and impact their overall quality of life. Below we will explore some strategies for managing sleep disturbances related to arthritis.

One of the most common sleep disturbances associated with arthritis is difficulty falling asleep or staying asleep. Pain, discomfort, and stiffness can make it challenging for individuals to get comfortable enough to fall asleep. It's essential to develop a consistent sleep routine that promotes relaxation and sleepiness. This could involve setting a regular bedtime and wake-up time, practicing relaxation techniques such as deep breathing, meditation, or yoga, and avoiding stimulating activities before bed, such as watching TV or using electronic devices.

For people who find it challenging to get comfortable enough to sleep, there are a few things that they can do to improve their sleep environment. For example, using a supportive mattress and pillow can help alleviate joint pain and pressure points. Some people may also find that using extra pillows to prop up painful joints or using a body pillow for support can be helpful. Additionally, keeping the bedroom cool, dark, and quiet can help create a relaxing sleep environment.

Another common sleep disturbance related to arthritis is waking up during the night due to pain or discomfort. In these instances, it can be helpful to have pain relief medication available and use it as needed. It's important to work with a healthcare provider to develop an effective pain management plan. There are also some non-pharmacological pain management techniques that can be helpful, such as heat therapy or topical creams.

Stress and anxiety can also contribute to sleep disturbances related to arthritis. The pain and limitations caused by arthritis can be emotionally distressing, which can make it difficult to relax and fall asleep. Practicing stress management techniques such as deep breathing, meditation, or visualization can help manage stress and anxiety. It may also be helpful to talk to a mental health professional who can provide support and guidance on coping with the emotional aspects of living with arthritis.

It's essential to remember that good sleep hygiene practices can help improve sleep quality and reduce sleep disturbances related to arthritis. Some general tips for good sleep hygiene include:

1. Creating a relaxing sleep environment: Make sure your bedroom is cool, dark, and quiet.

2. Establishing a consistent sleep routine: Go to bed and wake up at the same time every day, even on weekends.

3. Limiting stimulating activities before bed: Avoid using electronic devices or watching TV before bed.

4. Getting regular exercise: Exercise can help reduce pain and stiffness associated with arthritis and improve sleep quality.

5. Eating a healthy diet: Eating a healthy, balanced diet can help reduce inflammation and improve overall health.

6. Managing stress: Stress and anxiety can contribute to sleep disturbances. Managing stress through techniques like deep breathing, meditation, or visualization can help improve sleep quality.

In some cases, it may be necessary to consult a healthcare provider for further evaluation and treatment of sleep disturbances related to arthritis. They may recommend medications or other treatments to help manage sleep disturbances.

Chapter Twenty-Three

Arthritis and Weather Sensitivity

Arthritis is a chronic condition that affects millions of people worldwide. It is characterized by inflammation in the joints, leading to pain, stiffness, and reduced mobility. Although the exact cause of arthritis is still unknown, studies have shown that weather sensitivity is a significant factor that exacerbates arthritis symptoms. People with arthritis may experience increased pain and stiffness during changes in the weather, such as rainy days, cold temperatures, or high humidity.

Weather sensitivity in arthritis is a common phenomenon. It is believed that changes in temperature and humidity levels alter the pressure within the joints, leading to increased pain and discomfort. Barometric pressure changes, which occur before a storm, have also been associated with arthritis pain. The pressure drop can cause tissues around the joints to expand, leading to increased inflammation and pain. However, not everyone with arthritis is affected by weather sensitivity. Some people may not notice any difference in their symptoms, while others may experience severe pain and stiffness.

Managing weather sensitivity in arthritis requires a multi-faceted approach. One way to reduce the impact of weather on arthritis symptoms is to monitor the weather forecast and plan activities accordingly. For example, on days with cold or wet weather, people with arthritis should consider staying indoors or limiting their activities to those that are less strenuous. They may also choose to wear appropriate clothing, such as warm layers or waterproof shoes, to minimize exposure to the elements.

Maintaining a healthy lifestyle is another critical factor in managing arthritis and weather sensitivity. Regular exercise can help to strengthen the muscles and joints, reducing the risk of injury and easing arthritis pain. Low-impact exercises such as swimming, cycling, or yoga can be particularly effective. A balanced diet that includes plenty of fresh fruits and vegetables, lean proteins, and whole grains can also help to reduce inflammation and boost overall health.

In addition to lifestyle changes, various treatments can help manage weather sensitivity in arthritis. Pain medications such as nonsteroidal anti-inflammatory drugs (NSAIDs) and acetaminophen can help to reduce pain and inflammation. Topical creams and ointments that contain capsaicin or menthol can also provide temporary relief from arthritis pain.

Some people with arthritis may benefit from more advanced treatment options, such as corticosteroid injections or joint replacement surgery. Corticosteroid injections are a type of steroid medication that can be injected directly into the affected joint, providing immediate pain relief. Joint replacement surgery may be recommended for people with severe arthritis that has not responded to other treatments. During this procedure, the damaged joint is replaced with an artificial joint, improving mobility and reducing pain.

In addition to these traditional treatments, alternative therapies such as acupuncture, massage, and chiropractic care may also be effective in managing arthritis symptoms. These therapies work by targeting pressure points and reducing tension in the muscles and joints, providing relief from pain and stiffness.

Why some people are weather-sensitive

Many people with arthritis often report that changes in the weather can impact their pain and stiffness levels. In fact, studies have shown that changes in temperature, barometric pressure, and humidity can have a significant effect on arthritis symptoms. But why do some people experience weather sensitivity, while others do not?

Firstly, it's important to understand that the relationship between weather and arthritis symptoms is complex and not fully understood. However, researchers have proposed several theories on why some individuals may be more susceptible to weather changes than others.

One theory is that changes in atmospheric pressure can impact joint tissues. When atmospheric pressure drops, the tissues around the joints may expand, causing pressure and pain. Similarly, when the pressure rises, these tissues may contract, leading to stiffness and discomfort. This may explain why individuals with arthritis in weight-bearing joints, such as the hips and knees, may be more susceptible to weather sensitivity, as these joints are more affected by changes in pressure.

Another theory is that changes in temperature and humidity can affect nerve endings in the joints, leading to an increase in pain perception. Cold weather, in particular, can cause joint stiffness, making movement more difficult and painful. Humidity can also impact arthritis symptoms, as high levels of moisture in the air can cause swelling and inflammation in the joints.

Genetics may also play a role in weather sensitivity. Some individuals may have a genetic predisposition to arthritis and may be more sensitive to weather changes due to their genetic makeup. Additionally, individuals with certain types of arthritis, such as rheumatoid arthritis, may be more prone to weather sensitivity than those with osteoarthritis.

Finally, lifestyle factors may contribute to weather sensitivity in arthritis. For example, individuals who are less physically active or have a sedentary lifestyle may experience more joint pain and stiffness during changes in weather. Similarly, individuals who are overweight or obese may experience more pressure on their joints, exacerbating arthritis symptoms during weather changes.

Tips for coping with weather-related pain

Arthritis is a condition that affects millions of people worldwide. It is a chronic disease characterized by joint inflammation and pain, which can be exacerbated by various factors, including changes in weather. Weather changes can cause fluctuations in barometric pressure, humidity, and temperature, which can lead to increased joint pain and stiffness. These changes can be challenging to manage, but there are ways to cope with weather-related pain and minimize its impact on daily life.

One of the reasons why some people are more weather-sensitive than others is not entirely clear. However, it is known that changes in barometric pressure can affect the pressure inside joints, causing pain and discomfort. When barometric pressure drops, the tissues inside the joints may expand, leading to increased pressure and pain. Similarly, when the temperature drops, the tissues can contract, causing stiffness and pain. Humidity can also play a role in weather-related pain. High humidity levels can cause the tissues in the joints to swell, which can lead to pain and discomfort.

While there is no cure for arthritis, there are several ways to manage weather-related pain. The following are some tips for coping with weather-related pain:

1. Stay active: It may be tempting to avoid physical activity when experiencing joint pain. However, staying active is essential to maintaining

joint flexibility and strength. Exercise can also help improve overall health, which can reduce the severity of arthritis symptoms.

2. Stay warm: Cold temperatures can cause joint stiffness and pain. Dressing warmly and staying indoors during cold weather can help minimize these symptoms. It may also be helpful to use a heating pad or take a warm bath to ease joint pain.

3. Maintain a healthy weight: Excess weight can put additional stress on joints, leading to increased pain and discomfort. Maintaining a healthy weight can reduce the strain on joints and improve arthritis symptoms.

4. Use assistive devices: There are several assistive devices available that can help reduce joint pain and make daily tasks easier. These devices include canes, braces, and splints.

5. Practice relaxation techniques: Stress and anxiety can exacerbate arthritis symptoms. Practicing relaxation techniques, such as deep breathing, meditation, or yoga, can help reduce stress levels and improve overall health.

6. Consult a healthcare provider: A healthcare provider can help develop a personalized treatment plan to manage weather-related pain. This plan may include medications, physical therapy, or other interventions to manage arthritis symptoms.

7. Keep a diary: Keeping a diary of symptoms and weather changes can help identify patterns and triggers of weather-related pain. This information can be helpful in developing a management plan and communicating with healthcare providers.

Climate considerations for arthritis sufferers

Climate considerations for arthritis sufferers

Arthritis is a chronic condition that affects the joints, causing pain, stiffness, and reduced mobility. While there is no cure for arthritis, there are many ways to manage its symptoms, such as taking medication, exercising regularly, and making lifestyle changes. However, climate can also play a role in the management of arthritis, as certain weather conditions can exacerbate symptoms. Below we will discuss climate considerations for arthritis sufferers, including how weather affects arthritis and what steps can be taken to minimize its impact.

How weather affects arthritis

Many people with arthritis report that weather changes can affect their symptoms, causing increased pain and stiffness. The exact reasons for this are not yet fully understood, but there are several theories. One possibility is that changes in barometric pressure and humidity levels can affect the pressure inside joints, leading to pain and discomfort. Another theory is that cold weather can cause the muscles and tissues around the joints to tighten up, increasing pain and stiffness.

Whatever the cause, it is clear that weather changes can have a significant impact on arthritis symptoms. In fact, some studies have shown that up to 70% of arthritis sufferers are weather-sensitive, meaning that they experience increased pain and stiffness during certain weather conditions.

Climate considerations for arthritis sufferers

Given the impact that weather changes can have on arthritis symptoms, it is important for arthritis sufferers to take climate considerations into account when managing their condition. Here are some tips for managing arthritis symptoms in different climate conditions:

Hot weather:

For arthritis sufferers in hot climates, it is important to stay hydrated and cool. Make sure to drink plenty of water, wear loose-fitting clothing, and stay in air-conditioned spaces as much as possible. You may also want to avoid being outside during the hottest parts of the day, and plan outdoor activities for early morning or late evening when temperatures are cooler.

Cold weather:

For arthritis sufferers in cold climates, it is important to stay warm and keep your joints moving. Wear warm clothing, including gloves, hats, and scarves, and use heating pads or warm compresses to ease pain and stiffness. Exercise regularly to keep your joints flexible, but be sure to warm up first and avoid overexertion. You may also want to consider taking warm baths or using a sauna to relax your muscles and ease joint pain.

Humid weather:

For arthritis sufferers in humid climates, it is important to keep your joints as dry as possible. Wear moisture-wicking clothing and shoes, and use antiperspirant to reduce sweating. Stay in air-conditioned spaces as much as possible, and avoid being outside during the hottest and most humid parts of the day.

Dry weather:

For arthritis sufferers in dry climates, it is important to stay hydrated and moisturized. Drink plenty of water, and use lotion or other moisturizers to prevent dry skin and cracking around your joints. You may also want to use a humidifier to add moisture to the air inside your home.

Chapter Twenty-Four

Pregnancy and Arthritis

Pregnancy is a time of immense joy and excitement, but it can also be a time of stress and worry, particularly for women with arthritis. Arthritis is a chronic condition that causes inflammation in the joints, leading to pain, stiffness, and limited mobility. For women with arthritis, pregnancy can pose unique challenges, as they must balance the demands of pregnancy with the management of their arthritis symptoms. Below we will explore the impact of arthritis on pregnancy and provide tips for managing arthritis during pregnancy.

Arthritis and Pregnancy

Pregnancy can affect arthritis in different ways, depending on the type of arthritis a woman has. In some cases, pregnancy can lead to an improvement in arthritis symptoms, while in others, it can exacerbate symptoms.

For women with rheumatoid arthritis (RA), pregnancy can be a time of remission, as hormonal changes in the body can reduce inflammation in the joints. However, this improvement is not guaranteed, and some women with RA may experience increased symptoms during pregnancy. Additionally, women with RA who are pregnant may be at an increased risk of complications, such as preterm birth, preeclampsia, and gestational diabetes.

Women with osteoarthritis (OA), on the other hand, may experience increased symptoms during pregnancy, as the extra weight and pressure on the joints can exacerbate pain and stiffness. Furthermore, certain medications used to manage OA symptoms may not be safe during pregnancy, making it more challenging to manage symptoms.

Tips for Managing Arthritis During Pregnancy

If you have arthritis and are planning to become pregnant or are already pregnant, there are several strategies you can use to manage your symptoms and promote a healthy pregnancy. Here are some tips:

1. Work with your healthcare provider: Before trying to conceive, speak with your rheumatologist or obstetrician to discuss your plans and the potential impact of pregnancy on your arthritis. Your healthcare provider can help you determine the best course of action to manage your symptoms during pregnancy and ensure the safety of any medications you are taking.

2. Stay active: Regular exercise is important for maintaining joint health and reducing pain and stiffness. During pregnancy, low-impact exercises such as walking, swimming, and prenatal yoga can be helpful for managing arthritis symptoms. Be sure to speak with your healthcare provider before starting any new exercise regimen.

3. Practice self-care: Stress and anxiety can exacerbate arthritis symptoms, so it's important to prioritize self-care during pregnancy. This may include activities such as meditation, mindfulness, or massage therapy.

4. Use heat or cold therapy: Applying heat or cold to affected joints can help reduce pain and inflammation. A warm compress or heating pad can be used to relax stiff joints, while a cold compress or ice pack can help reduce swelling and inflammation.

5. Consider physical therapy: Physical therapy can be a helpful tool for managing arthritis during pregnancy. A physical therapist can develop

an individualized exercise program to help improve joint flexibility and mobility.

6. Seek emotional support: Dealing with chronic pain and a chronic condition can be stressful and emotionally draining. Seeking support from friends, family, or a mental health professional can help you cope with the challenges of arthritis and pregnancy.

Managing arthritis during pregnancy

Managing arthritis during pregnancy can be a challenge for women who suffer from this chronic condition. Arthritis is a group of conditions that cause joint pain and inflammation, affecting millions of people worldwide. Pregnancy, on the other hand, is a unique time that comes with its own set of challenges. When a woman is pregnant, she needs to take care of herself and her growing baby while managing her arthritis symptoms.

There are several types of arthritis, and each requires different management strategies during pregnancy. Rheumatoid arthritis (RA), psoriatic arthritis, and lupus are three common types of arthritis that can affect women during pregnancy.

Rheumatoid arthritis is a chronic autoimmune disease that causes inflammation in the joints, leading to pain and stiffness. During pregnancy, RA can improve for some women, while it worsens for others. Many women with RA report feeling better during pregnancy due to increased levels of hormones, such as estrogen and progesterone. However, some women may experience flare-ups during the postpartum period.

Psoriatic arthritis is another form of arthritis that can affect women during pregnancy. This condition causes joint pain, swelling, and stiffness, as well as skin symptoms such as red, scaly patches on the skin. Women with psoriatic arthritis may experience a worsening of symptoms during pregnancy, particularly in the later stages. Treatment options for psoriatic arthritis during pregnancy may include corticosteroids, nonsteroidal anti-inflammatory drugs (NSAIDs), and disease-modifying antirheumatic drugs (DMARDs).

Lupus is a chronic autoimmune disease that can cause inflammation and damage to various parts of the body, including the joints, skin, kidneys, and heart. Women with lupus may be at higher risk for pregnancy complications, such as pre-eclampsia, miscarriage, and preterm birth. Managing lupus during pregnancy may require close monitoring by a healthcare provider and adjustments to medications.

It is essential for women with arthritis to work closely with their healthcare providers to manage their condition during pregnancy. The goal is to maintain disease control while minimizing any potential risks to the developing baby.

There are several strategies that women with arthritis can use to manage their condition during pregnancy. These include:

1. Staying active: Regular exercise can help reduce joint pain and stiffness while improving overall physical and mental health. Low-impact activities such as walking, swimming, and prenatal yoga are safe options for pregnant women.

2. Maintaining a healthy diet: A balanced diet rich in fruits, vegetables, lean protein, and whole grains can help reduce inflammation and improve overall health.

3. Getting enough rest: Getting enough sleep and taking breaks throughout the day can help reduce fatigue and manage arthritis symptoms.

4. Using hot or cold therapy: Applying a heating pad or cold pack to affected joints can help reduce pain and inflammation.

5. Practicing stress management techniques: Stress can worsen arthritis symptoms, so practicing relaxation techniques such as deep breathing, meditation, or guided imagery can help manage stress and reduce symptoms.

6. Taking medications as prescribed: Women with arthritis should work with their healthcare providers to develop a medication plan that is safe for both them and their developing baby.

7. Seeking emotional support: Living with a chronic condition such as arthritis can be challenging, and pregnancy can add additional stress. Seeking support from friends, family, or a therapist can help manage emotions and improve mental health.

Medications and pregnancy safety

Medications and Pregnancy Safety in Arthritis Management

Arthritis is a common condition that affects millions of people worldwide. It is characterized by joint pain, stiffness, and swelling that can significantly affect a person's quality of life. While there are many ways to manage arthritis symptoms, including lifestyle changes, physical therapy, and medications, pregnancy can complicate the management of arthritis. During pregnancy, many women are concerned about the safety of the medications they take to manage their arthritis symptoms. Below we will discuss the safety of arthritis medications during pregnancy and offer some tips for managing arthritis during pregnancy.

1. Arthritis medications are classified into four main categories: non-steroidal anti-inflammatory drugs (NSAIDs), disease-modifying an-

tirheumatic drugs (DMARDs), biologic response modifiers, and corticosteroids. NSAIDs are commonly used to reduce inflammation and pain in arthritis, while DMARDs are used to modify the course of the disease. Biologic response modifiers are a newer class of drugs that target specific parts of the immune system that are involved in arthritis. Corticosteroids are potent anti-inflammatory drugs that are often used in the short-term to manage arthritis symptoms.

Many of these medications are not considered safe during pregnancy, particularly in the first trimester when fetal organs are developing. Some NSAIDs, such as ibuprofen and naproxen, have been linked to an increased risk of miscarriage and birth defects. DMARDs, such as methotrexate, can cause fetal abnormalities and should not be used during pregnancy. Biologic response modifiers are also not recommended during pregnancy due to their potential to harm the developing fetus. Corticosteroids are generally considered safe in pregnancy, but high doses or long-term use may increase the risk of pregnancy complications.

So, what options do pregnant women with arthritis have for managing their symptoms? Fortunately, there are many non-medication options available. These include physical therapy, heat and cold therapy, acupuncture, and exercise. These non-medication options can be effective at reducing inflammation and pain, without the risk of harming the developing fetus.

For women who must continue to take arthritis medications during pregnancy, there are some steps that can be taken to minimize the risks. First, it is essential to talk to your doctor about the risks and benefits of continuing the medication. Some women may need to switch to a safer medication during pregnancy, while others may be able to continue taking their current medication. Second, it is essential to take the medication as directed and only at the recommended dose. Taking more medication than prescribed can increase the risk of side effects. Finally, it is essential to attend all prenatal appointments and notify your doctor of any changes in your condition or symptoms.

It is also important to remember that pregnancy can affect arthritis symptoms. Many women experience an improvement in arthritis symptoms during pregnancy, particularly in the second trimester. However, some women may experience a worsening of their symptoms during pregnancy. This is due to the changes in hormone levels and increased stress on the joints.

Postpartum arthritis care

Postpartum arthritis is a type of arthritis that occurs after childbirth. It can be a challenging condition to manage, particularly for new mothers who may also be dealing with the demands of caring for a newborn. Below we will discuss the causes, symptoms, and treatment options for postpartum arthritis, as well as strategies for managing the condition.

Postpartum arthritis can occur in women who have previously been diagnosed with rheumatoid arthritis or another autoimmune disease, as well as those who have never experienced arthritis symptoms before. The hormonal changes that occur during pregnancy can lead to a temporary suppression of the immune system, which can cause a flare-up of arthritis symptoms after delivery. Additionally, the physical stress of childbirth and the demands of caring for a newborn can exacerbate joint pain and inflammation.

Symptoms of postpartum arthritis can include joint pain, stiffness, and swelling. The symptoms may be most severe in the first few months after delivery, but they can persist for several months or even years. Women with postpartum arthritis may experience difficulty with everyday activities such as dressing, carrying their baby, or lifting objects.

Treatment options for postpartum arthritis are similar to those for other types of arthritis. Nonsteroidal anti-inflammatory drugs (NSAIDs) such as ibuprofen or naproxen can help relieve pain and inflammation. Corticosteroids may be prescribed for more severe symptoms, but they should be used with caution due to the potential for side effects. Disease-modifying antirheumatic drugs (DMARDs) such as methotrexate or sulfasalazine may be used in cases where NSAIDs and corticosteroids are not effective.

In addition to medication, there are several strategies that women with postpartum arthritis can use to manage their symptoms. Physical therapy can help improve joint mobility and strength, and can also provide guidance on safe exercise during the postpartum period. Occupational therapy can help women adapt to their new roles as mothers and develop strategies for completing everyday tasks despite joint pain or stiffness.

Another important aspect of managing postpartum arthritis is self-care. This may include getting adequate rest, practicing stress-management techniques, and maintaining a healthy diet. Women with postpartum arthritis may also find it helpful to use assistive devices such as splints, braces, or crutches to reduce joint stress and pain.

It is important for women with postpartum arthritis to communicate with their healthcare providers about their symptoms and treatment options. Women who are breastfeeding should discuss medication options with their providers, as some medications may not be safe for nursing infants. Providers can also offer support and guidance on coping with the emotional challenges of living with arthritis while caring for a newborn.

Chapter Twenty-Five

Arthritis and Intimacy

Arthritis is a chronic condition that can affect all aspects of a person's life, including their intimate relationships. It is estimated that approximately one-third of people with arthritis report experiencing sexual problems related to their condition. These issues can include pain, fatigue, decreased mobility, and medication side effects, all of which can affect a person's ability to engage in sexual activity and intimacy.

One of the main concerns for people with arthritis is pain. Joint pain can make sexual positions uncomfortable or even impossible, and sexual activity can also cause pain and stiffness in the affected joints. Additionally, fatigue and decreased mobility can make it difficult for people with arthritis to engage in prolonged sexual activity. Medications used to manage arthritis symptoms can also affect sexual function, with some causing erectile dysfunction or decreased libido.

It is important for people with arthritis to talk to their healthcare providers about their sexual health concerns. Treatment options for arthritis-related sexual problems can include pain management strategies, physical therapy, and medication adjustments. Couples can also work together to find sexual positions and activities that are comfortable and enjoyable for both partners.

In addition to physical challenges, arthritis can also affect a person's emotional and mental well-being, which can impact their intimate relationships. Depression, anxiety, and stress can all contribute to sexual problems, as well as feelings of low self-esteem and a lack of sexual confidence.

It is important for people with arthritis to prioritize their mental health and seek support when needed. This can include therapy, support groups, and self-care activities such as meditation, exercise, and relaxation techniques. Talking openly with a partner about emotional concerns and sexual challenges can also help to strengthen the relationship and improve intimacy.

There are also several products and devices available that can help people with arthritis to engage in sexual activity comfortably. For example, sex pillows and supports can provide additional support and reduce joint pain during sexual activity. Lubricants can also help to reduce friction and increase comfort during sexual activity.

It is important to note that intimacy is not solely defined by sexual activity. Non-sexual forms of intimacy such as cuddling, hugging, and kissing can also be an important part of a relationship. Couples can work together to find alternative forms of physical connection and intimacy that are comfortable and enjoyable for both partners.

Navigating the challenges of intimacy

Arthritis is a condition that affects millions of people around the world, and it can have a significant impact on various aspects of their lives, including their intimate relationships. Arthritis can cause chronic pain, fatigue, and stiffness, which can make it challenging to engage in sexual activity. Additionally, the emotional toll of living with a chronic condition can lead to feelings of anxiety, depression, and self-consciousness, which can also affect intimacy. However, there are ways to navigate the challenges of intimacy when living with arthritis.

The first step is to communicate openly and honestly with your partner. It can be challenging to talk about the impact that arthritis has on your body and your sex life, but it's essential to have an open dialogue. This can help you both understand each other's needs and limitations and find ways to adapt and adjust to make sex more comfortable and enjoyable. Try to approach the conversation with a positive and collaborative attitude, and be willing to listen to your partner's perspective and needs.

It's also essential to explore different positions and techniques that can help alleviate pain and discomfort. Experimenting with different positions can help you find ones that work best for your body. For example, lying on your side with a pillow between your knees can alleviate pressure on your hips and lower back. Using cushions or pillows to support your body can also help to reduce pain and fatigue. Additionally, trying different forms of sexual activity, such as massage or manual stimulation, can help to maintain intimacy while reducing pain.

Using assistive devices can also be helpful when managing arthritis during intimacy. For example, using a sex pillow can provide support and reduce pressure on your joints during sex. A lubricant can also help to reduce friction and discomfort. If you're experiencing vaginal dryness due to arthritis medication or other factors, consider using a water-based lubricant to make sex more comfortable. If you have mobility issues, you may want to consider using a bed rail or other support device to make getting in and out of bed easier.

It's also essential to prioritize self-care and manage arthritis symptoms outside of the bedroom. This can include practicing stress-reducing techniques like meditation, yoga, or deep breathing exercises, as stress can exacerbate arthritis symptoms. Additionally, eating a healthy diet, getting regular exercise, and getting enough sleep can all help to manage arthritis symptoms and improve overall health.

Finally, it's important to seek support from healthcare professionals and arthritis support groups. A rheumatologist can help to manage your arthritis symptoms and may be able to recommend treatments that can improve your quality of life. Additionally, arthritis support groups can provide a safe and supportive environment to discuss issues related to arthritis and intimacy.

Tips for maintaining a healthy sex life

Arthritis can have a significant impact on one's physical and emotional health, including their sex life. However, with the right strategies and mindset, individuals with arthritis can still maintain a healthy and fulfilling sex life. Below we will discuss some tips for maintaining a healthy sex life despite arthritis.

First and foremost, communication is key. It is essential to talk openly and honestly with your partner about your condition and how it may impact your sexual activities. This can include discussing what positions and movements are most comfortable, as well as any other concerns or limitations that may arise. Being open and transparent with your partner can help alleviate any anxieties or misunderstandings, and can ultimately lead to a more enjoyable and satisfying sexual experience.

Secondly, taking care of oneself is crucial. This includes managing pain and discomfort through medication, exercise, or other therapies, as well as maintaining a healthy diet and lifestyle. A healthy body and mind can lead to increased confidence and comfort in sexual situations.

It is also important to explore alternative forms of sexual expression. This can include experimenting with different positions or sexual acts that may be more comfortable and less painful. Additionally, incorporating other forms of intimacy such as kissing, cuddling, or massage can also be a great way to connect with your partner and maintain a healthy sexual relationship.

Furthermore, using aids and devices such as pillows, wedges, or vibrators can help alleviate discomfort and enhance pleasure. There are many devices on the market specifically designed for individuals with arthritis, such as ergonomic sex toys and special pillows to support joints and reduce pain.

Another important factor in maintaining a healthy sex life is maintaining an open and positive attitude towards sex. Arthritis can often lead to feelings of depression, anxiety, and low self-esteem, which can negatively impact one's sexual desire and enjoyment. However, by actively working to cultivate a positive and confident mindset towards sex, individuals with arthritis can continue to enjoy intimacy and connection with their partner.

Finally, seeking support from a healthcare professional or support group can be beneficial. A healthcare professional can provide guidance on pain management, medication, and other treatments that may help alleviate arthritis symptoms and improve sexual function. Additionally, a support group can provide a safe and understanding environment to discuss personal concerns and challenges related to arthritis and sexuality.

Communicating with your partner

Arthritis is a chronic condition that can affect many aspects of a person's life, including their intimate relationships. The pain, stiffness, and fatigue associated with arthritis can make sexual activity difficult or uncomfortable, and it can also cause emotional stress and strain on relationships. It is important for those with arthritis to communicate with their partners openly and honestly about their condition and to work together to find ways to maintain a healthy and fulfilling sex life.

One of the challenges of arthritis and intimacy is the physical limitations that can come with the condition. Arthritis pain and stiffness can make it difficult to move or change positions during sexual activity, and it can also make certain positions more uncomfortable or even impossible. Fatigue can also be a factor, as arthritis can cause exhaustion and reduce energy levels. These physical limitations can be frustrating and can lead to a decrease in sexual activity or avoidance altogether.

To overcome these challenges, it is important to find ways to adapt sexual activity to make it more comfortable and enjoyable. Experimenting with different positions, using pillows or other props for support, and taking breaks when needed can all help to make sex more comfortable and enjoyable. It is also important to prioritize rest and relaxation, both before and after sexual activity, to help reduce fatigue and improve energy levels.

Another challenge of arthritis and intimacy is the emotional impact it can have on relationships. Arthritis can cause feelings of frustration, embarrassment, or shame, and it can be difficult to talk about these feelings with a partner. It is important for those with arthritis to communicate openly and honestly with their partners about their feelings and to seek support when needed.

One way to improve communication about arthritis and intimacy is to seek counseling or therapy. A therapist can help individuals and couples to navigate the emotional challenges of arthritis and to find ways to improve communication and intimacy. It is also important to be patient and understanding with each other, and to recognize that arthritis is a chronic condition that can have a significant impact on a person's life.

There are also a number of practical tips that can help to maintain a healthy sex life with arthritis. For example, using lubricants can help to reduce discomfort and improve sexual pleasure, while practicing relaxation techniques, such as deep breathing or meditation, can help to reduce stress and tension. It is also important to stay active and maintain a healthy weight, as this can help to reduce arthritis symptoms and improve overall health.

In addition to these tips, it is important to talk to a healthcare provider about any concerns related to arthritis and intimacy. A healthcare provider can provide guidance on managing arthritis symptoms, including pain management, and can also offer advice on safe and effective sexual practices.

Chapter Twenty-Six

Arthritis and Your Feet

Arthritis is a condition that affects millions of people worldwide. It is a chronic inflammatory disease that affects the joints and can cause pain, stiffness, and swelling. One of the most common areas affected by arthritis is the feet. The feet are vital for mobility and balance, and arthritis can make it challenging to perform daily activities. Below we will discuss arthritis in the feet and how to manage it effectively.

There are several types of arthritis that can affect the feet, including osteoarthritis, rheumatoid arthritis, and gout. Osteoarthritis is the most common type of arthritis, and it is caused by the wear and tear of cartilage in the joints. Rheumatoid arthritis is an autoimmune disease that affects the joints, and gout is caused by the buildup of uric acid crystals in the joints.

Arthritis in the feet can cause a range of symptoms, including pain, swelling, stiffness, and reduced mobility. The pain can be particularly severe in the morning or after periods of inactivity. Arthritis in the feet can also cause deformities, such as bunions, hammertoes, and flat feet.

Managing arthritis in the feet requires a multifaceted approach that includes medication, exercise, and lifestyle changes. Nonsteroidal anti-inflammatory drugs (NSAIDs) are commonly used to reduce pain and inflammation. In severe cases, corticosteroid injections may be necessary. Physical therapy can help improve mobility and reduce pain. Exercises that strengthen the muscles around the feet and ankles can also help alleviate symptoms.

Lifestyle changes can also help manage arthritis in the feet. Wearing comfortable shoes that provide support and cushioning can help reduce pressure on the joints. Orthotic devices, such as shoe inserts, can also provide additional support and cushioning. Maintaining a healthy weight can also help reduce the strain on the feet and joints.

There are also several home remedies that can help alleviate symptoms of arthritis in the feet. Applying ice packs or heating pads to the affected area can help reduce pain and inflammation. Epsom salt baths can also help reduce pain and stiffness. Foot massages and stretching exercises can help improve flexibility and reduce pain.

In addition to these treatments, there are also several surgeries that can help manage arthritis in the feet. Joint replacement surgery is a common treatment for severe cases of arthritis. This involves replacing the damaged joint with an artificial one. Arthrodesis is another surgical option that fuses the affected joint together.

Preventing arthritis in the feet is possible by maintaining a healthy weight, wearing comfortable shoes, and avoiding high-impact activities that can cause damage to the joints. Regular exercise, such as walking or swimming, can also help maintain joint health.

Types of arthritis affecting the feet

Arthritis is a condition characterized by inflammation and pain in the joints. While many people associate arthritis with the hands or knees, it can affect any joint in the body, including the feet. The feet are complex structures, consisting of many bones, joints, and ligaments. When arthritis affects the feet, it can cause significant pain and disability, making it difficult to walk or engage in daily activities.

There are several types of arthritis that can affect the feet, including:

1. Osteoarthritis: This is the most common type of arthritis, and it occurs when the protective cartilage that covers the ends of bones wears down over time. When this happens in the feet, it can cause pain, stiffness, and swelling.

2. Rheumatoid arthritis: This is an autoimmune disorder in which the body's immune system attacks the joints, causing inflammation and damage. Rheumatoid arthritis can affect any joint in the body, including those in the feet.

3. Gout: This is a type of arthritis that occurs when uric acid crystals build up in the joints, causing inflammation and pain. Gout often affects the big toe, causing it to become red, swollen, and painful.

4. Psoriatic arthritis: This is a type of arthritis that occurs in people with psoriasis, a skin condition characterized by red, scaly patches. Psoriatic arthritis can affect the feet, causing pain, swelling, and stiffness.

5. Ankylosing spondylitis: This is a type of arthritis that primarily affects the spine, but it can also affect the feet. Ankylosing spondylitis can cause pain and stiffness in the feet, making it difficult to walk.

Regardless of the type of arthritis that affects the feet, the symptoms are often similar. These include:

Pain, stiffness, and swelling in the feet

Difficulty walking or standing for long periods

Reduced range of motion in the feet and ankles

Numbness or tingling in the feet

Deformities in the joints of the feet

If you are experiencing any of these symptoms, it is important to see a doctor for an accurate diagnosis and treatment plan.

Treatment for arthritis in the feet typically involves a combination of medication, physical therapy, and lifestyle changes. Nonsteroidal anti-inflammatory drugs (NSAIDs) can help reduce pain and inflammation, while disease-modifying antirheumatic drugs (DMARDs) may be used to slow the progression of the disease. Physical therapy can help improve mobility and reduce pain, while lifestyle changes such as weight loss and exercise can help improve overall health and reduce the impact of arthritis on the feet.

In some cases, surgery may be necessary to treat arthritis in the feet. This may involve joint replacement surgery or fusion surgery to stabilize the joint and reduce pain.

Proper foot care and footwear

Arthritis can affect any joint in the body, including the feet. In fact, the feet are particularly vulnerable to arthritis because they support the body's weight and are subjected to a great deal of stress and impact during daily activities. Arthritis in the feet can cause pain, stiffness, and limited mobility, making it difficult to perform even the simplest tasks. Fortunately, there are steps you can take to manage your foot arthritis and improve your overall foot health.

The first step in managing foot arthritis is to understand the type of arthritis you have. There are several types of arthritis that can affect the feet, including osteoarthritis, rheumatoid arthritis, and gout. Osteoarthritis is the most common form of arthritis and is caused by wear and tear on the joints over time. Rheumatoid arthritis is an autoimmune disease that causes inflammation and damage to the joints. Gout is a form of arthritis that occurs when uric acid crystals accumulate in the joints, causing pain and inflammation.

Once you know the type of arthritis you have, you can work with your healthcare provider to develop a treatment plan. Depending on the severity of your condition, treatment options may include medications, physical therapy, or surgery. In addition to medical treatment, there are also several things you can do to improve your foot health and manage your arthritis symptoms.

One of the most important things you can do to manage foot arthritis is to take good care of your feet. This includes keeping your feet clean and dry, trimming your toenails regularly, and wearing shoes that fit properly and provide adequate support. Shoes that are too tight or too loose can put extra pressure on your joints and exacerbate arthritis symptoms. Look for shoes that have a wide toe box, good arch support, and a cushioned sole. Avoid high heels, which can increase the pressure on the balls of your feet.

Orthotic devices can also be helpful in managing foot arthritis. Orthotics are specially designed shoe inserts that provide additional support and cushioning to the feet. They can help distribute your weight more evenly and reduce the stress on your joints. There are many different types of orthotics available, and your healthcare provider can help you choose the one that is best for your needs.

In addition to taking care of your feet and wearing proper footwear, there are also exercises you can do to improve foot arthritis symptoms. Strengthening exercises can help improve the stability and function of your feet, while stretching exercises can help improve flexibility and reduce stiffness. Your healthcare provider or a physical therapist can recommend exercises that are appropriate for your condition and help you develop a safe and effective exercise plan.

Managing foot arthritis can be challenging, but with proper care and treatment, it is possible to reduce pain and improve mobility. If you are experiencing foot pain or stiffness, it is important to talk to your healthcare provider and get an accurate diagnosis. With the right treatment plan and lifestyle changes, you can take control of your foot arthritis and improve your overall quality of life.

Orthotic devices and supports

Arthritis is a condition that affects the joints and can cause inflammation, pain, and stiffness. It can also affect the feet, making it difficult to walk and perform daily activities. Orthotic devices and supports can help manage foot pain and improve mobility for people with arthritis.

Orthotic devices are specialized shoe inserts designed to provide additional support and cushioning to the foot. They can help redistribute pressure and alleviate pain caused by arthritis. Orthotics are available in a range of materials, including foam, plastic, and silicone. They can be customized to fit the individual foot, providing the best possible support and comfort.

One common type of orthotic device is an arch support. Arch supports help support the foot's arch and can reduce pain caused by flat feet or fallen arches. They can also help prevent the foot from rolling inward, which can cause pain and discomfort.

Another type of orthotic device is a heel cup. Heel cups are designed to cushion and support the heel, reducing pressure and pain in the foot. They can also help correct any alignment issues that may be causing pain.

In addition to orthotic devices, supportive shoes can also be helpful for people with arthritis. Shoes with a wide toe box can provide more room for the toes and reduce pressure on the foot. Shoes with a cushioned sole can also help reduce shock and pressure when walking.

When choosing shoes, it's important to find a pair that fits well and provides adequate support. Shoes that are too tight or too loose can cause discomfort and increase the risk of foot injuries. Shoes should also be chosen based on the individual's level of activity. For example, someone who enjoys walking should choose a supportive walking shoe, while someone who plays sports may need a specialized athletic shoe.

Foot supports can also be used to provide additional support and cushioning. Toe supports can help alleviate pain caused by hammertoes or other toe deformities. Ankle supports can help stabilize the ankle and reduce the risk of sprains or other injuries.

Finally, exercises and stretches can help improve foot strength and flexibility, reducing the risk of foot injuries and managing arthritis symptoms. Exercises that focus on stretching and strengthening the feet, such as toe curls and ankle rotations, can be helpful. Yoga and Pilates can also be beneficial, as they focus on improving flexibility and balance.

Chapter Twenty-Seven

Arthritis in Pets

Arthritis is a common health condition that affects millions of people around the world, but did you know that it can also affect our beloved pets? Arthritis in pets can be just as painful and debilitating as it is in humans, and it can significantly impact their quality of life. Below we will discuss what arthritis in pets is, its causes, symptoms, and how it can be managed.

Arthritis in pets is a degenerative joint disease that causes inflammation and damage to the joints. It is also known as osteoarthritis, and it is most commonly seen in older pets, although younger animals can also be affected. Arthritis can occur in any joint in the body, but it is most commonly seen in the hips, knees, elbows, and spine.

There are several factors that can contribute to the development of arthritis in pets. One of the most common causes is simply aging. As pets get older, the cartilage in their joints breaks down, leading to inflammation and pain. Other factors that can contribute to the development of arthritis include obesity, genetics, trauma to the joints, and certain underlying medical conditions.

The symptoms of arthritis in pets can vary depending on the severity of the condition and the location of the affected joint. Some common symptoms include limping or favoring one leg, stiffness, difficulty getting up or lying down, reluctance to walk or play, and irritability or aggression when touched. In some cases, pets may also develop a fever or lose their appetite.

If you suspect that your pet may be suffering from arthritis, it is important to seek veterinary care right away. Your vet will perform a physical examination and may also recommend X-rays or other diagnostic tests to confirm the diagnosis. Once the diagnosis has been made, your vet will work with you to develop a treatment plan that is tailored to your pet's needs.

The goal of treatment for arthritis in pets is to relieve pain and inflammation, as well as to slow the progression of the disease. There are several different types of treatment that may be recommended, depending on the severity of the condition. In some cases, simple changes to your pet's diet or exercise routine may be enough to manage their symptoms. In other cases, medication may be necessary to reduce pain and inflammation. Surgery may also be an option in severe cases.

In addition to traditional treatments, there are also several alternative therapies that may be helpful in managing arthritis in pets. These can include acupuncture, massage, hydrotherapy, and the use of supplements such as glucosamine and chondroitin. It is important to discuss any alternative therapies with your veterinarian before trying them, to ensure that they are safe and effective for your pet.

Another important aspect of managing arthritis in pets is providing them with a comfortable and supportive living environment. This can include providing them with a soft, supportive bed, ramps or stairs to help them navigate their home, and non-slip flooring to prevent falls. It is also important to keep your pet at a healthy weight, as excess weight can put extra stress on their joints and make their symptoms worse.

Recognizing arthritis in pets

Arthritis is a common condition that affects millions of people worldwide, but did you know that it can also affect pets? Yes, you read that right! Arthritis is not exclusive to humans, and it can cause discomfort and pain in our furry companions as well. While arthritis in pets can be challenging to diagnose, it is essential to recognize the symptoms to provide them with the care they need. Below we will discuss how to recognize arthritis in pets and what steps pet owners can take to help their pets live comfortably.

Arthritis, also known as osteoarthritis, is a degenerative joint disease that occurs when the cartilage between the bones wears away, causing the bones to rub against each other, leading to pain, inflammation, and stiffness. Arthritis is most commonly seen in dogs, especially those who are middle-aged or older, overweight, or have had previous joint injuries. Cats can also develop arthritis, but it is less common in cats than dogs.

One of the most common signs of arthritis in pets is limping or favoring one leg over another. Pets may also appear stiff when getting up after sleeping or have difficulty jumping up or down from high places like furniture. They may also avoid certain activities they once enjoyed, such as running or playing. You may also notice your pet licking or chewing on a particular area, indicating pain or discomfort in that area. It is essential to pay attention to these signs and seek veterinary care if necessary.

There are many things pet owners can do to help their furry companions with arthritis. The first step is to take your pet to the vet for a proper diagnosis. Your veterinarian can provide a treatment plan that is tailored to your pet's specific needs, which may include medications, supplements, and lifestyle changes.

One way to manage arthritis in pets is through exercise. Exercise can help strengthen the muscles around the affected joint, providing support and reducing pain. However, it is essential to choose low-impact activities that do not put a lot of strain on the joints. Activities such as walking, swimming, or gentle stretching can be beneficial.

Another way to manage arthritis in pets is through weight management. Pets who are overweight are more likely to develop arthritis and are more likely to experience pain and discomfort. It is essential to maintain a healthy weight and provide your pet with a balanced diet that is rich in nutrients.

Supplements such as glucosamine and chondroitin can also be helpful in managing arthritis in pets. These supplements can help repair and strengthen cartilage, reducing pain and inflammation in the affected joints. It is essential to talk to your veterinarian before starting any supplements, as they can interact with other medications.

Orthotic devices and supports can also be beneficial in managing arthritis in pets. These devices can help provide support to the affected joint, reducing pain and inflammation. Examples of orthotic devices include braces, splints, and wraps. However, it is essential to consult with your veterinarian before using any orthotic devices.

Treatment options for pets

Arthritis is not a condition that only affects humans; it is a common problem in pets, especially in dogs and cats. Arthritis in pets can be caused by various factors, including age, weight, genetics, and previous injuries. Just like in humans, arthritis in pets can be a painful and debilitating condition that affects their quality of life. However, with proper diagnosis and treatment, pets with arthritis can live long and comfortable lives. Below we will discuss the various treatment options available for pets with arthritis.

Medications

One of the most common treatment options for arthritis in pets is medication. Just like in humans, there are different types of medications available for pets with arthritis. Some of the most common medications used to treat arthritis in pets include non-steroidal anti-inflammatory drugs (NSAIDs), corticosteroids, and disease-modifying anti-rheumatic drugs (DMARDs).

NSAIDs are commonly used to manage the pain and inflammation associated with arthritis in pets. Some of the commonly used NSAIDs for pets include carprofen, meloxicam, and firocoxib. However, it is important to note that long-term use of NSAIDs can have some side effects, such as gastrointestinal problems, liver damage, and kidney damage.

Corticosteroids, such as prednisone and dexamethasone, are also commonly used to manage the inflammation associated with arthritis. However, these medications can also have side effects, such as increased thirst and appetite, weight gain, and increased risk of infection.

DMARDs are another class of medications that are commonly used to manage arthritis in pets. These medications work by slowing down the progression of the disease, and they are commonly used for pets with rheumatoid arthritis. Some of the commonly used DMARDs for pets include methotrexate and leflunomide.

Supplements

Supplements are another popular treatment option for pets with arthritis. Some of the commonly used supplements for pets with arthritis include glucosamine, chondroitin, and omega-3 fatty acids.

Glucosamine and chondroitin are commonly used to improve joint health and reduce inflammation in pets with arthritis. These supplements work by promoting the production of cartilage in the joints, which helps to improve joint health and mobility.

Omega-3 fatty acids are also commonly used to manage the inflammation associated with arthritis in pets. These supplements are known for their anti-inflammatory properties, and they have been shown to reduce joint pain and stiffness in pets with arthritis.

Physical therapy and exercise

Physical therapy and exercise can also be used to manage arthritis in pets. These treatment options are especially useful for pets with mild to moderate arthritis. Physical therapy can help to improve joint mobility and reduce joint pain, while exercise can help to improve muscle strength and reduce weight, which can help to reduce the pressure on the joints.

Some of the common physical therapy options for pets with arthritis include massage therapy, hydrotherapy, and cold laser therapy. These treatments can help to reduce joint pain and inflammation and improve joint mobility.

Exercise is also important for pets with arthritis. However, it is important to choose low-impact exercises that do not put too much strain on the joints. Some of the common exercises for pets with arthritis include walking, swimming, and gentle stretching exercises.

Surgery

In some cases, surgery may be necessary to manage arthritis in pets. Surgery is usually recommended for pets with severe arthritis that is not responding to other treatment options. Some of the common surgical options for pets with arthritis include joint replacement surgery and joint fusion surgery.

Joint replacement surgery involves replacing the damaged joint with an artificial joint. This surgery is usually recommended for pets with severe joint damage that cannot be repaired through other treatment options.

Joint fusion surgery involves fusing the

Supporting your pet's quality of life

Arthritis is not just a human condition, it can also affect our furry friends. In fact, arthritis is one of the most common ailments in pets, affecting millions of cats and dogs worldwide. As pet owners, it is important to recognize the signs of arthritis and provide the necessary support to improve their quality of life.

The first step in supporting your pet's quality of life is to recognize the signs of arthritis. Pets are good at hiding pain, so it is important to be observant and proactive. Some of the most common signs of arthritis in pets include limping, difficulty walking, reluctance to climb stairs or jump up on furniture, and a decrease in overall activity level. You may also notice changes in your pet's personality, such as increased irritability or withdrawal.

If you suspect that your pet has arthritis, it is important to consult with your veterinarian. Your vet can diagnose arthritis and recommend treatment options based on the severity of your pet's condition. Treatment options may include medication, supplements, and physical therapy.

Medications are often the first line of treatment for pets with arthritis. Nonsteroidal anti-inflammatory drugs (NSAIDs) are commonly used to reduce inflammation and alleviate pain. However, these medications can have side effects, so it is important to closely monitor your pet and follow your vet's instructions.

In addition to medication, supplements may also be recommended to support your pet's joint health. Glucosamine and chondroitin are commonly used to promote cartilage health, while omega-3 fatty acids can reduce inflammation and improve joint mobility.

Physical therapy can also be beneficial for pets with arthritis. Exercise can help improve joint mobility and reduce pain. Your vet may recommend specific exercises for your pet or refer you to a physical therapist who specializes in pet rehabilitation.

It is also important to make adjustments to your pet's environment to support their mobility. Providing ramps or steps can make it easier for your pet to climb up and down furniture or navigate stairs. Soft bedding can also help alleviate pressure on their joints.

Finally, it is important to provide emotional support for your pet. Arthritis can be a frustrating and painful condition, and your pet may become irritable or withdrawn. Spending quality time with your pet, providing toys and activities that they enjoy, and giving plenty of positive reinforcement can help improve their mood and overall quality of life.

Chapter Twenty-Eight

Cooking and Arthritis

1. Cooking and Arthritis: Tips and Strategies for Managing Joint Pain in the Kitchen

Arthritis is a chronic condition that affects millions of people worldwide, and one of its most challenging aspects is managing daily activities such as cooking. Arthritis can cause pain, stiffness, and reduced range of motion, making it difficult to handle pots and pans, chop ingredients, and perform other kitchen tasks. However, with some modifications and adaptations, it is possible to continue cooking and enjoying delicious meals despite arthritis. This article will discuss tips and strategies for managing joint pain in the kitchen.

Understanding the Challenges

Before diving into the strategies, it's essential to understand the challenges that arthritis presents in the kitchen. Arthritis can affect various joints in the body, including the hands, wrists, elbows, and shoulders, making it challenging to perform basic tasks like chopping vegetables or opening jars. Arthritis can also cause fatigue, making it difficult to stand for extended periods or carry heavy objects. The symptoms of arthritis can also be aggravated by temperature changes or repetitive motions, both of which are common in the kitchen. Cooking can be frustrating, but it doesn't have to be impossible.

Adapting Your Kitchen

One of the first steps to managing arthritis in the kitchen is adapting the space to make it more accessible and comfortable. Here are some ideas to consider:

2. Install pull-out shelves: These can help you avoid reaching into deep cabinets, which can strain your shoulders and neck.

3. Use a lazy susan: This rotating platform can be helpful for accessing spices or other small items that are stored in a corner cabinet.

4. Install a lever-handle faucet: This type of faucet is easier to operate than traditional knobs, which can be difficult to turn if you have hand arthritis.

5. Use a cart or trolley: A kitchen cart or trolley can provide additional counter space and storage, making it easier to move heavy pots and pans around the kitchen.

6. Use lightweight cookware: Non-stick pans, aluminum pots, and other lightweight cookware can be easier to handle than heavy cast iron or stainless steel.

7. Install drawer organizers: Drawer organizers can make it easier to find utensils and other kitchen tools quickly.

Modifying Cooking Techniques

Once you've adapted your kitchen space, the next step is to modify your cooking techniques. Here are some tips to consider:

8. Use a food processor: A food processor can make it easier to chop vegetables and other ingredients, saving time and reducing strain on your hands.

9. Use an electric can opener: An electric can opener is easier to operate than a manual one, which can be difficult to turn if you have hand arthritis.

10. Use a jar opener: A jar opener can help you open stubborn lids without straining your wrists or fingers.

11. Avoid repetitive motions: Try to vary your movements and avoid performing the same motion repeatedly, which can cause joint pain and fatigue.

12. Take breaks: If you're cooking for an extended period, take breaks to rest your joints and reduce fatigue.

13. Use adaptive tools: There are many adaptive tools available, such as angled utensils, specialized cutting boards, and easy-grip handles, that can make cooking easier and more comfortable.

Healthy Eating for Arthritis

In addition to modifying your kitchen space and cooking techniques, it's essential to focus on healthy eating to manage arthritis. Here are some dietary tips to consider:

14. Focus on anti-inflammatory foods: Arthritis is an inflammatory condition, so it's important to eat foods that can help reduce inflammation. Examples include leafy greens, fatty fish, nuts, and berries.

15. Limit processed foods: Processed foods are often high in sugar, salt, and unhealthy fats, which can contribute to inflammation and joint pain.

16. Stay hydrated: Drinking plenty of water

Adapting your kitchen for arthritis

Adapting your kitchen for arthritis is an important step towards making everyday tasks easier and less painful. Arthritis can make simple tasks like cooking a meal or preparing snacks more difficult, and the kitchen can be a hazardous place for those with joint pain or limited mobility. However, with some modifications to your kitchen, you can make cooking and meal preparation easier and safer.

The first step in adapting your kitchen for arthritis is to evaluate your current setup. Take a look at your kitchen and think about what tasks are most challenging for you. This may include reaching for items in high cabinets, opening jars, or standing for long periods of time. Once you have identified the areas that need improvement, you can begin making modifications to your kitchen.

One important modification is to make sure that your kitchen is well-lit. Good lighting is important for people with arthritis because it can help them see what they are doing and reduce the risk of falls. Install task lighting over the stove and countertops to make it easier to see what you are doing.

Another modification is to adjust the height of your countertops and work surfaces. This can be done by adding a raised cutting board or using a kitchen island with an adjustable height. This will make it easier to work in the kitchen without having to bend over or strain your back.

You may also want to consider adding pull-out shelves or drawers to your cabinets. This will make it easier to reach items in the back of the cabinets without having to stretch or bend over. Lazy Susans and turntables can also be useful for accessing items that are difficult to reach.

When it comes to cooking utensils and tools, there are many options available that are designed specifically for people with arthritis. Look for tools with easy-grip handles, such as rubber or silicone grips, to reduce the strain on your hands and wrists. Electric can openers, jar openers, and other kitchen tools can also be helpful in reducing the amount of effort required to complete a task.

If standing for long periods of time is difficult, consider adding a stool or chair to your kitchen. This will allow you to take breaks as needed and reduce the strain on your feet and legs. A cushioned mat can also be helpful for reducing the impact on your joints while standing.

Finally, consider using kitchen appliances that make cooking easier and require less physical effort. Slow cookers, rice cookers, and pressure cookers can all be helpful for reducing the amount of time spent standing over a hot stove. Microwaves and toaster ovens can also be useful for heating up small meals or snacks without having to use the stove.

Adapting your kitchen for arthritis can make a big difference in your daily life. By making modifications to your kitchen, you can reduce the amount of pain and discomfort associated with cooking and meal preparation. Talk to your doctor or a physical therapist for more tips on how to make your kitchen arthritis-friendly.

Cooking techniques for arthritis sufferers

Arthritis is a condition that can cause pain, stiffness, and inflammation in the joints. These symptoms can make everyday tasks, such as cooking, challenging for those who suffer from the condition. However, with some adjustments to cooking techniques, those with arthritis can still enjoy preparing and eating delicious, nutritious meals.

One of the key considerations for those with arthritis is minimizing stress on the joints. This can be achieved by choosing lightweight cookware, such as aluminum or ceramic pots and pans, which are easier to handle than heavy cast-iron cookware. Handles on cookware should also be large and ergonomic, to make them easier to grip and reduce the strain on the hands and wrists.

In addition to choosing the right cookware, modifying the cooking process itself can also make a big difference. For example, rather than standing for long periods of time stirring a pot, it may be easier to use a slow cooker or pressure cooker that requires less attention. These devices can help simplify the cooking process and reduce the need for constant monitoring.

Another helpful technique for arthritis sufferers is to use kitchen tools and gadgets that are specifically designed to reduce joint stress. For example, an electric can opener can be much easier to use than a manual one, and a food processor can make chopping and dicing ingredients much quicker and easier. Similarly, using a jar opener or a rubber grip pad can make opening jars and bottles much less of a strain on the hands and wrists.

When it comes to cutting and chopping ingredients, using a specialized cutting board can make a big difference. A cutting board with a non-slip surface can help reduce the risk of slips and falls, while a cutting board with a raised lip can help keep ingredients from spilling onto the countertop. Some cutting boards are also designed to be used at an angle, which can reduce the strain on the wrists and hands.

When it comes to preparing and cooking meals, there are also some general tips that can be helpful for those with arthritis. For example, taking breaks to stretch and move around can help reduce stiffness and fatigue, and avoiding repetitive motions can help prevent strain on the joints. It is also important to pace oneself and not take on too much at once, as this can lead to overexertion and increased pain and fatigue.

In addition to modifying cooking techniques and using specialized tools and gadgets, there are also some dietary changes that may be helpful for those with arthritis. For example, consuming foods that are high in omega-3 fatty acids, such as fatty fish and nuts, may help reduce inflammation in the body. Similarly, avoiding processed foods, refined sugars, and excessive amounts of saturated fat may also be beneficial.

Meal planning and preparation tips

Meal planning and preparation can be a challenge for anyone, but for those with arthritis, it can be especially difficult. Arthritis can cause pain, stiffness, and limited mobility in the hands, making it hard to chop vegetables, lift pots, and perform other cooking tasks. However, with some adjustments and tips, it is possible to continue enjoying home-cooked meals.

One key to successful meal planning and preparation is to make the kitchen as accessible and user-friendly as possible. This may involve making some modifications to the kitchen, such as installing pull-out shelves, lowering countertops, or replacing traditional knobs with easier-to-grip handles.

In addition, using adaptive equipment can make cooking much easier for those with arthritis. This might include items such as jar openers, cutting boards with built-in clamps, or kitchen shears with spring-loaded handles. These types of tools can make chopping, slicing, and opening jars much less painful and challenging.

When it comes to meal planning, it can be helpful to plan ahead and prepare meals in advance whenever possible. This might involve setting aside some time each week to chop vegetables, cook grains, and prepare other ingredients that can be used in a variety of meals. Having pre-cooked ingredients on hand can make it much easier to put together healthy, home-cooked meals even on days when arthritis symptoms are particularly troublesome.

Another option is to make use of kitchen gadgets that can speed up the cooking process. A slow cooker, for example, can be a great way to prepare healthy meals with minimal hands-on time. Simply load up the slow cooker in the morning with ingredients like meat, vegetables, and spices, and let it cook all day while you go about your other tasks.

For those who find meal planning and preparation to be especially challenging, there are many meal delivery services that specialize in providing healthy, home-cooked meals to those with specific health conditions like arthritis. These services can take the stress and hassle out of meal planning and preparation, while still providing healthy and delicious meals that meet your nutritional needs.

Finally, it is important to remember that cooking and meal planning should not be a source of stress or anxiety. If you are finding it too difficult to prepare meals on your own, it is okay to ask for help from family members or friends, or to consider using one of the many resources available to make meal planning and preparation easier.

Chapter Twenty-Nine

Gardening and Arthritis

Gardening is a wonderful hobby that provides physical exercise, mental relaxation, and the joy of growing your own fruits, vegetables, and flowers. However, for individuals with arthritis, the physical demands of gardening can be challenging. Arthritis is a condition that causes joint pain and stiffness, which can make gardening difficult. Despite these challenges, with a few modifications and adjustments, gardening can still be a enjoyable and rewarding hobby for people with arthritis.

Arthritis is a common condition that affects millions of people worldwide. There are over 100 different types of arthritis, with osteoarthritis and rheumatoid arthritis being the most common. Osteoarthritis is caused by the wear and tear of joints over time, while rheumatoid arthritis is an autoimmune disease that causes joint inflammation.

Gardening requires a range of movements, including bending, kneeling, reaching, and lifting. These movements can put a strain on the joints and exacerbate arthritis symptoms. However, there are several modifications and adjustments that can be made to help reduce the strain on the joints.

Firstly, it is important to choose the right tools. There are several ergonomic tools available that are designed to reduce the strain on the joints. For example, long-handled tools can help reduce the need for bending and reaching, while tools with padded handles can provide a more comfortable grip. Additionally, using lightweight tools can help reduce the strain on the joints when lifting and carrying.

Secondly, it is important to use proper techniques. For example, using a wheelbarrow or garden cart to transport heavy items can help reduce the strain on the joints. Additionally, using raised garden beds or containers can help reduce the need for bending and kneeling. Using a stool or chair to sit on while gardening can also help reduce the strain on the joints.

Thirdly, it is important to take frequent breaks. Gardening can be physically demanding, and it is important to take breaks to rest and stretch. It is recommended to take a break every 20-30 minutes to stretch and relax the joints.

Fourthly, it is important to listen to your body. If you experience pain or discomfort while gardening, it is important to take a break and rest the affected joints. It is also important to avoid overexertion and to pace yourself throughout the gardening session.

Lastly, it is important to engage in regular exercise and physical activity to help maintain joint flexibility and strength. Engaging in low-impact exercises such as swimming, cycling, or yoga can help improve joint flexibility and reduce the symptoms of arthritis.

In addition to these modifications and adjustments, there are also several gardening activities that are particularly well-suited for individuals with arthritis. For example, container gardening allows individuals to garden from a seated position, reducing the need for bending and kneeling. Additionally, planting small herbs and vegetables in pots can be a great way to enjoy the benefits of gardening without the physical demands of larger-scale gardening.

Another activity that is well-suited for individuals with arthritis is flower arranging. This activity involves arranging flowers in vases or other containers and can be done indoors or outdoors. Flower arranging is a creative and relaxing activity that does not require the physical demands of traditional gardening.

Benefits of gardening for arthritis sufferers

Gardening is a hobby enjoyed by many people around the world. It is a great way to get outside and enjoy the fresh air while also being active and productive. For those who suffer from arthritis, gardening can be especially beneficial. Arthritis is a condition that causes inflammation in the joints, which can be painful and limit mobility. However, gardening can help alleviate some of these symptoms and provide a range of other benefits for arthritis sufferers.

One of the main benefits of gardening for arthritis sufferers is that it is a low-impact form of exercise. It can be a great way to stay active and maintain joint flexibility without putting too much strain on the joints. Gardening can involve a range of activities, from digging and planting to weeding and pruning. These movements can help improve joint mobility and reduce stiffness.

In addition to providing physical benefits, gardening can also have positive effects on mental health. Spending time in nature and tending to plants has been shown to reduce stress and promote relaxation. For arthritis sufferers who may experience anxiety or depression due to their condition, gardening can be a helpful tool for improving mental health and well-being.

Another benefit of gardening for arthritis sufferers is the opportunity to grow fresh produce. Eating a healthy and balanced diet is important for managing arthritis symptoms and maintaining overall health. By growing their own fruits and vegetables, arthritis sufferers can ensure they are consuming fresh and nutrient-rich foods.

However, gardening can be challenging for those with arthritis, as it can involve a lot of bending, kneeling, and reaching. Fortunately, there are several adaptations and techniques that can make gardening easier and more comfortable for arthritis sufferers. Here are some tips for arthritis sufferers who want to enjoy gardening:

1. Use raised garden beds: Raised garden beds can be a great solution for arthritis sufferers, as they allow for gardening without having to bend down or kneel. They can also be designed to fit any height or size, making them customizable to individual needs.

2. Use ergonomic tools: Ergonomic gardening tools are designed to be easier on the hands and joints, reducing strain and discomfort. Look for tools with padded handles, long handles, or specialized shapes that make them easier to grip.

3. Take breaks: It is important to take regular breaks when gardening to avoid overexertion and fatigue. Set a timer to remind yourself to take a break every 30 minutes or so, and use this time to stretch and rest.

4. Use a garden stool or kneeler: A garden stool or kneeler can provide a comfortable and supportive surface for gardening. These tools can help reduce strain on the knees and back, making gardening more comfortable and enjoyable.

5. Use raised container gardens: Raised container gardens can be a great alternative to traditional gardens, especially for those with limited space. They can be placed on patios, decks, or balconies, and can be customized to fit individual needs and preferences.

Adapting your garden for arthritis

Arthritis can make everyday tasks difficult, including gardening, which may seem like a challenging activity for those who suffer from this condition. However, with some adaptations, gardening can become a therapeutic and enjoyable hobby for arthritis sufferers. Below we will discuss how to adapt your garden for arthritis and make it an accessible and enjoyable activity.

The first step to adapting your garden for arthritis is to create a suitable workspace. A raised garden bed is an excellent option for those with arthritis as it allows you to garden at a comfortable height without having to bend or kneel. Raised garden beds can be purchased, or you can build one yourself using bricks, stones, or lumber. The ideal height for a raised garden bed is between 18 and 24 inches, making it easy to reach without straining your back or joints. Additionally, consider installing a sturdy handrail or railing near your garden bed to provide support when standing up or sitting down.

Another option to consider is container gardening. This is a great way to garden if you have limited space or mobility. Container gardening allows you to plant and care for a variety of plants, herbs, and vegetables in pots or containers of different sizes and shapes. Container gardening can be done indoors or outdoors and is an excellent option for those with arthritis who have limited mobility.

Choosing the right tools for gardening is also crucial when adapting your garden for arthritis. Look for lightweight and ergonomic tools that are easy to grip and maneuver. Long-handled tools such as a hoe or cultivator can help you avoid bending and kneeling, while hand tools such as pruners or secateurs can help you easily cut through branches and stems without straining your hands. Additionally, consider investing in a gardening stool or bench that provides support and allows you to work at a comfortable height.

One of the most critical aspects of gardening with arthritis is pacing yourself. Start with short sessions and gradually increase the duration of your gardening as your stamina improves. Avoid overworking yourself and take breaks when you need to. If you feel pain or discomfort, stop gardening and rest your joints. Applying a cold or warm compress to your joints can also help relieve pain and inflammation.

Another important consideration when adapting your garden for arthritis is choosing plants that are easy to maintain and care for. Look for low-maintenance plants that require minimal watering, pruning, or deadheading. Consider planting herbs, succulents, or other plants that require minimal upkeep. Avoid plants with thorns, prickly leaves, or branches, which can be difficult to handle and may cause injury.

In addition to adapting your garden, it is also essential to practice good self-care when gardening with arthritis. Wearing protective gear such as gloves, long sleeves, and a hat can protect your skin from the sun and prevent scratches or cuts. Staying hydrated and taking breaks when needed can also help you avoid overexertion and fatigue. Furthermore, consider using a topical pain reliever or taking over-the-counter pain medication to manage pain and inflammation.

Finally, it is essential to consult with your doctor or healthcare provider before starting any new activity, including gardening. They can help you determine what modifications may be necessary and provide guidance on how to manage your arthritis while gardening. Additionally, they can provide recommendations on pain management and assistive devices such as braces or supports that may help alleviate joint pain.

Gardening tools and techniques for arthritis

Gardening can be an enjoyable and rewarding hobby for people of all ages. However, for those who suffer from arthritis, gardening can become a challenge due to joint pain and stiffness. Arthritis is a condition that affects the joints and causes inflammation, swelling, and pain. It is a chronic condition that can affect people's mobility and their ability to perform everyday tasks, including gardening.

Fortunately, there are several ways to adapt gardening techniques and tools to make it possible for people with arthritis to continue to enjoy their gardening hobby.

Firstly, selecting the right tools for the job is essential for people with arthritis. Long-handled tools with soft-grip handles can reduce strain on the hands and wrists. Tools with padded handles are also a good option for those who suffer from arthritis pain in their hands. Ergonomic tools are specially designed to reduce the strain on the body, making gardening more comfortable for people with arthritis.

Secondly, creating raised beds or container gardens is another option for gardeners with arthritis. Raised garden beds can be built at a height that is comfortable for the gardener, reducing the need for bending and kneeling. Container gardens can also be placed at a height that is comfortable for the gardener and can be moved around to suit changing weather conditions.

Thirdly, planning ahead is essential for gardeners with arthritis. Scheduling gardening tasks for times when joints are least painful, such as during the morning or on a cool day, can make a big difference in how comfortable gardening is. Breaking up tasks into smaller, more manageable parts and taking frequent breaks can also help to prevent joint pain and stiffness.

Fourthly, gardening techniques can be adapted to be more arthritis-friendly. For example, using a lightweight hose instead of a heavy watering can

can reduce the strain on the arms and shoulders. Using a garden kneeler or padded stool can also make it more comfortable to work at ground level.

Fifthly, warming up before gardening is essential for people with arthritis. Gentle stretching exercises before gardening can help to improve joint mobility and reduce the risk of injury. Cold packs or heat pads can also be used to reduce joint pain and stiffness after gardening.

Finally, it is important for people with arthritis to listen to their bodies and to seek help when needed. If a task is causing excessive pain or discomfort, it is important to take a break or to ask for help from a family member or friend. It is also essential to consult a healthcare professional if arthritis symptoms are worsening or if new symptoms develop.

Chapter Thirty

Self-Care and Mindfulness

Self-care and mindfulness are two powerful tools that can help people with arthritis manage their symptoms and improve their overall well-being. Arthritis is a chronic condition that can cause pain, stiffness, and inflammation in the joints, making it difficult to perform daily tasks and enjoy life. While there is no cure for arthritis, there are many ways to manage the condition and reduce its impact on daily life. Self-care and mindfulness are two approaches that can be used to complement medical treatment and promote physical and emotional health.

Self-care refers to activities that people can do to take care of their physical, mental, and emotional health. For people with arthritis, self-care may involve exercise, eating a healthy diet, getting enough sleep, and taking time to rest and recharge. Exercise is an important component of self-care for people with arthritis because it can help reduce pain and stiffness, increase range of motion, and improve overall fitness. Low-impact activities such as walking, swimming, and cycling are good choices for people with arthritis because they are easy on the joints. Strength training exercises can also be helpful for building muscle and protecting the joints.

In addition to exercise, self-care for people with arthritis may involve making dietary changes to reduce inflammation and improve overall health. Eating a diet that is rich in fruits, vegetables, whole grains, lean protein, and healthy fats can provide the nutrients that the body needs to function properly and may help reduce inflammation. Avoiding foods that are high in sugar, saturated fat, and processed ingredients may also be helpful in managing arthritis symptoms.

Another important component of self-care is getting enough rest and taking time to relax. For people with arthritis, getting enough sleep can help reduce pain and stiffness and improve overall health. Practicing relaxation techniques such as deep breathing, meditation, and yoga can also be helpful in reducing stress and promoting a sense of calm.

Mindfulness is another approach that can be used to help manage arthritis symptoms and improve overall well-being. Mindfulness involves paying attention to the present moment and accepting one's thoughts and feelings without judgment. Mindfulness practices such as meditation, guided imagery, and body scans can help reduce stress, anxiety, and depression, which are common in people with arthritis.

Studies have shown that mindfulness can be helpful in reducing pain and improving quality of life in people with arthritis. Mindfulness practices can help people with arthritis become more aware of their thoughts and feelings and develop a greater sense of control over their condition. Mindfulness can also help people with arthritis cultivate a sense of compassion and acceptance, which can promote emotional well-being and reduce stress.

In addition to mindfulness practices, self-compassion can also be an important component of self-care for people with arthritis. Self-compassion involves treating oneself with kindness and understanding, rather than self-criticism and judgment. For people with arthritis, self-compassion may involve acknowledging the challenges of living with a chronic condition and giving oneself permission to rest and take care of oneself.

Self-care and mindfulness are powerful tools that can help people with arthritis manage their symptoms and improve their overall well-being. By incorporating self-care practices such as exercise, healthy eating, and rest into daily life, and cultivating mindfulness and self-compassion, people with arthritis can develop a greater sense of control over their condition and improve their quality of life. While there is no cure for arthritis, there are many ways to manage the condition and reduce its impact on daily life.

The role of self-care in arthritis management

Arthritis is a chronic condition that affects millions of people worldwide. It can cause inflammation and pain in the joints, making it difficult to perform daily activities. While there are various treatments available to manage arthritis symptoms, self-care plays a vital role in ensuring a better quality of life for those living with this condition.

Self-care refers to any activity or practice that an individual does to improve their physical, emotional, or mental health. In the case of arthritis, self-care can help manage symptoms and reduce pain, stiffness, and inflammation. Here are some of the ways self-care can be beneficial for people living with arthritis:

1. Exercise: Regular exercise can help strengthen muscles, improve joint flexibility, and reduce pain and stiffness associated with arthritis. Low-impact exercises like walking, cycling, and swimming are excellent options for people with arthritis, as they are gentle on the joints. It is important to speak with a healthcare professional before starting any exercise program to ensure it is safe and effective.

2. Healthy Diet: A healthy diet can help reduce inflammation and improve overall health. Foods that are rich in antioxidants, omega-3 fatty acids, and vitamin D, such as leafy greens, fatty fish, and nuts, can be particularly beneficial for people with arthritis.

3. Stress Management: Chronic stress can worsen arthritis symptoms. Activities like meditation, yoga, and deep breathing exercises can help reduce stress and promote relaxation.

4. Rest: Getting enough rest is important for managing arthritis symptoms. Adequate sleep can help reduce pain and inflammation and improve overall mood and energy levels.

5. Pain Management: Over-the-counter pain medications, such as acetaminophen and nonsteroidal anti-inflammatory drugs (NSAIDs), can help manage pain associated with arthritis. However, it is important to speak with a healthcare professional before taking any medication.

6. Joint Protection: Protecting joints is essential for managing arthritis symptoms. Simple changes like using assistive devices, such as canes or braces, and avoiding repetitive motions or activities that put excessive strain on the joints, can help prevent further damage.

In addition to these self-care practices, mindfulness techniques can also be beneficial for people living with arthritis. Mindfulness involves being fully present in the moment and accepting any sensations, emotions, or thoughts that arise without judgment.

Mindfulness techniques, such as deep breathing exercises, visualization, and progressive muscle relaxation, can help reduce stress and anxiety, which can exacerbate arthritis symptoms. These techniques can also help increase self-awareness and improve overall emotional and mental well-being.

Mindfulness practices for coping with pain

Arthritis is a chronic condition that affects millions of people around the world. It causes joint pain, stiffness, and swelling, and can significantly impact one's daily life. Although medication and physical therapy can help manage symptoms, practicing mindfulness techniques can also be beneficial for those living with arthritis. Mindfulness is a type of meditation that involves focusing on the present moment and accepting one's thoughts and feelings without judgment. Below we will explore the role of mindfulness practices in coping with arthritis pain.

One of the most common symptoms of arthritis is pain, which can be both physical and emotional. Mindfulness practices can help manage this pain by allowing individuals to become more aware of their thoughts and feelings related to the pain. By becoming more mindful, individuals can learn to observe their pain without judgment and become more accepting of it. This can help reduce stress and anxiety associated with the pain, which can in turn reduce the severity of the pain.

There are several mindfulness practices that can be helpful for coping with arthritis pain. One such practice is deep breathing, which involves taking slow, deep breaths and focusing on the sensations of the breath moving in and out of the body. This can help calm the mind and reduce stress and tension in the body. Another practice is body scanning, which involves paying attention to each part of the body and noticing any sensations or tension. By becoming more aware of the body, individuals can learn to identify areas of tension and work on releasing it through relaxation techniques.

Meditation is another mindfulness practice that can be helpful for managing arthritis pain. Meditation involves sitting quietly and focusing on the present moment, allowing thoughts and feelings to come and go without judgment. This can help individuals become more aware of their thoughts and feelings related to their pain, and develop a more accepting and compassionate attitude towards themselves. It can also help reduce stress and anxiety, which can exacerbate arthritis symptoms.

Yoga is another mindfulness practice that can be helpful for individuals with arthritis. Yoga involves a series of postures and movements, which can help increase flexibility and reduce stiffness in the joints. It can also help strengthen the muscles surrounding the joints, which can help provide additional support and reduce pain. By practicing yoga regularly, individuals can learn to become more mindful of their bodies and develop a more accepting and compassionate attitude towards themselves.

In addition to mindfulness practices, self-care is also an important aspect of managing arthritis. This includes getting adequate rest, eating a healthy diet, and engaging in regular physical activity. It also includes taking time for oneself, engaging in activities that bring joy and fulfillment, and seeking support from loved ones and healthcare professionals. By taking care of oneself, individuals can reduce stress and anxiety, which can exacerbate arthritis symptoms.

Relaxation techniques for stress relief

Relaxation techniques are often recommended for individuals with arthritis as a way to manage pain and reduce stress. Arthritis is a chronic condition that affects the joints, causing pain, stiffness, and limited mobility. It can also impact an individual's mental health and lead to increased stress and anxiety. Therefore, incorporating relaxation techniques into an arthritis management plan can be beneficial for both physical and mental well-being.

One relaxation technique that has been shown to be effective for individuals with arthritis is deep breathing exercises. Deep breathing involves taking slow, deep breaths in through the nose and out through the mouth. This technique can help to reduce stress and anxiety by slowing down the heart rate and promoting relaxation. Deep breathing can also help to reduce pain by increasing oxygen flow to the body, which can reduce inflammation.

Another relaxation technique that can be helpful for individuals with arthritis is progressive muscle relaxation. This technique involves tensing and relaxing different muscle groups in the body, one at a time. By doing so, individuals can become more aware of the sensations in their body and release tension that may be contributing to pain or discomfort. Progressive muscle relaxation can also help to reduce stress and promote relaxation, leading to a more restful sleep.

Meditation is another relaxation technique that has been shown to be effective for individuals with arthritis. Meditation involves focusing on a particular thought, object, or activity to promote mental clarity and relaxation. It can also help to reduce stress and anxiety, leading to improved mental and physical well-being. There are several types of meditation, including mindfulness meditation, which involves focusing on the present moment, and transcendental meditation, which involves repeating a mantra.

In addition to relaxation techniques, there are several other strategies that can be helpful for managing stress and anxiety related to arthritis. One such strategy is exercise. Exercise can help to improve joint function, reduce pain, and increase overall mobility. It can also promote relaxation and reduce stress by releasing endorphins, which are natural painkillers that promote a sense of well-being.

Another strategy for managing stress and anxiety related to arthritis is to engage in activities that bring joy and happiness. This may include hobbies, spending time with loved ones, or engaging in creative pursuits. By doing so, individuals can reduce stress and improve their overall quality of life.

Finally, it is important for individuals with arthritis to seek support from friends, family, or healthcare professionals. Support can help individuals to cope with the challenges of living with arthritis and provide them with the resources they need to manage their condition effectively.

Chapter Thirty-One

Arthritis and Creativity

Arthritis is a condition that affects the joints and can cause pain, stiffness, and inflammation. It is a common condition, with millions of people suffering from it worldwide. While arthritis can be a debilitating condition that can affect daily activities, there are ways to manage the symptoms and improve overall quality of life. One way to do this is through creativity.

Creativity is the ability to use imagination to come up with ideas, solutions, and expressions that are unique and original. It is a way to express oneself and to cope with stress and anxiety. Studies have shown that engaging in creative activities can have a positive impact on mental health, which is why it is increasingly being used as a form of therapy.

For people with arthritis, engaging in creative activities can be especially beneficial. Arthritis can limit mobility and cause pain, which can make daily tasks challenging. Engaging in creative activities can help distract from pain and provide a sense of purpose and accomplishment.

There are many ways to incorporate creativity into daily life for arthritis sufferers. Some examples include:

1. Painting and Drawing: Painting and drawing can be therapeutic for arthritis sufferers, as it provides a way to express emotions and feelings that may be difficult to put into words. It is also a low-impact activity that can be done from a seated position.

2. Crafting: Crafting can be a fun and creative way to keep the mind and hands busy. There are many different types of crafts that can be done, including knitting, crochet, and scrapbooking.

3. Writing: Writing can be a powerful way to express oneself and to cope with difficult emotions. It can also be a way to document one's experiences with arthritis, which can be helpful in managing the condition.

4. Music: Listening to music or playing a musical instrument can be a great way to relax and unwind. It can also provide a sense of accomplishment and boost self-esteem.

5. Photography: Photography is a creative hobby that can be done from a seated position. It can be a way to capture and document special moments and experiences.

Engaging in creative activities can also help improve overall mental health and well-being. It can reduce stress, anxiety, and depression, which are common comorbidities of arthritis. Studies have shown that creative activities can stimulate the brain and improve cognitive function, which is important for maintaining mental sharpness and preventing cognitive decline.

In addition to engaging in creative activities, there are other self-care practices that arthritis sufferers can incorporate into their daily routine. These include:

6. Exercise: Exercise is important for maintaining joint health and mobility. It can also help reduce pain and inflammation associated with arthritis.

7. Healthy Diet: Eating a healthy, balanced diet is important for overall health and well-being. It can also help manage symptoms of arthritis, as certain foods can exacerbate inflammation.

8. Rest and Relaxation: Rest and relaxation are essential for managing arthritis symptoms. It is important to get enough sleep and to take breaks throughout the day to rest and recharge.

9. Stress Management: Managing stress is important for overall health and well-being. Stress can exacerbate arthritis symptoms and increase inflammation in the body.

10. Support Groups: Joining a support group can provide a sense of community and support. It can also be a way to learn from others and to share experiences and strategies for managing arthritis.

The therapeutic benefits of creativity

The power of creativity is often underestimated, but it can be an incredibly valuable tool in managing chronic conditions like arthritis. Engaging in creative activities can have numerous benefits, including reducing stress and anxiety, promoting mindfulness and relaxation, and providing a sense of accomplishment and fulfillment. Below we will explore the therapeutic benefits of creativity for individuals with arthritis and how incorporating creative practices into their routine can enhance their overall well-being.

One of the most significant benefits of creativity for arthritis sufferers is the ability to reduce stress and anxiety. Chronic pain can cause individuals to feel overwhelmed, anxious, and depressed. Participating in creative activities can help alleviate these negative emotions by shifting the focus from pain to the present moment. For instance, painting, drawing, or writing can serve as an outlet to express emotions, providing a sense of relief from pain and reducing anxiety. Studies have shown that participating in creative activities can significantly reduce cortisol levels, the hormone that causes stress, and lower heart rate, leading to a sense of calmness and relaxation.

Another way that creativity can benefit individuals with arthritis is by promoting mindfulness and relaxation. Engaging in creative activities like knitting or coloring can provide an opportunity to focus on the present moment and quiet the mind. These activities can serve as a form of meditation, helping individuals to tune out the distractions of everyday life and focus on the task at hand. This can help to reduce stress and anxiety, improve concentration, and promote a sense of calmness.

Creativity can also provide individuals with arthritis a sense of accomplishment and fulfillment. Chronic pain can make it challenging to participate in everyday activities and accomplish simple tasks, leading to feelings of helplessness and frustration. Engaging in creative activities can provide a sense of purpose and accomplishment, even if it is just finishing a small project. This can boost self-esteem and provide a sense of control over one's life, leading to improved mood and overall well-being.

Incorporating creative practices into an individual's routine can take many forms. For example, individuals can start with simple activities such as coloring or knitting, which can be done while sitting and do not require a lot of energy. As individuals become more comfortable with creative activities, they can try more challenging projects like painting, writing, or pottery. Additionally, there are several group programs specifically designed for individuals with arthritis, like art therapy or music therapy, which can provide a supportive community and help individuals to connect with others who share similar experiences.

It is essential to note that creativity should not be used as a substitute for medical treatment but rather as a complementary therapy. Individuals should consult with their healthcare provider before starting any new activity or exercise program, especially if they have limitations due to their arthritis.

Adapting your creative practice for arthritis

Arthritis can present significant challenges to individuals who engage in creative activities such as painting, playing an instrument, or knitting. The pain, stiffness, and limited mobility that are common symptoms of arthritis can make it difficult to pursue these hobbies, leading to frustration and a decrease in quality of life. However, with the right strategies, it is possible to adapt your creative practice to better suit your needs and continue enjoying the therapeutic benefits of creative expression.

The first step in adapting your creative practice for arthritis is to identify the specific challenges you face. For example, if you experience pain and stiffness in your hands, you may struggle to hold a paintbrush or manipulate knitting needles. If you have arthritis in your back, you may find it uncomfortable to sit or stand for long periods while playing an instrument or working on a pottery wheel. Once you have a clear understanding of your limitations, you can start exploring ways to modify your practice to make it more accessible.

One effective strategy for adapting your creative practice is to invest in specialized equipment designed for individuals with arthritis or other mobility challenges. For example, there are ergonomic paintbrushes and crochet hooks that are designed to be more comfortable to hold and use for extended periods. There are also a variety of assistive devices available, such as grip aids and jar openers, that can make it easier to manipulate tools and materials.

Another approach to adapting your creative practice for arthritis is to modify your technique. For example, if you typically use a tight grip when holding a paintbrush, you may want to experiment with using a looser grip or holding the brush in a different way to reduce strain on your hands.

Similarly, you may be able to modify the way you hold an instrument or adjust your posture to reduce discomfort.

In addition to modifying your equipment and technique, it can be helpful to adjust the way you approach your creative practice. For example, you may find it more comfortable to break up your painting sessions into shorter, more manageable periods rather than attempting to complete an entire painting in one sitting. You could also experiment with different types of materials or projects that require less fine motor control or physical exertion. Ultimately, the goal is to find a way to engage in creative expression that is enjoyable and fulfilling without causing undue pain or discomfort.

It is worth noting that adapting your creative practice for arthritis may require a certain degree of trial and error. It may take some time to find the right combination of equipment, technique, and approach that works for you. It is also important to be patient and to take breaks as needed to avoid exacerbating your symptoms. Remember that the goal is not perfection but rather to find a way to continue pursuing your creative passions in a way that is comfortable and sustainable.

In addition to the practical benefits of adapting your creative practice for arthritis, there are also numerous therapeutic benefits to engaging in creative expression. Studies have shown that creative activities such as painting, music, and knitting can help to reduce stress and anxiety, improve mood, and boost overall well-being. For individuals with arthritis, who may be at increased risk for depression and other mental health challenges, engaging in creative activities can be a valuable tool for promoting emotional and psychological resilience.

Finding inspiration and motivation

Arthritis can be a challenging condition to manage, but finding ways to stay inspired and motivated can make a big difference. One way to do this is through finding inspiration and motivation in creative pursuits, such as art, writing, music, and more.

Creativity has long been known to have therapeutic benefits, both for mental and physical health. Studies have shown that engaging in creative activities can help reduce stress, anxiety, and depression, as well as improve cognitive function and overall wellbeing.

For those with arthritis, creative pursuits can also help manage pain and improve mobility. By focusing on an activity that brings joy and fulfillment, individuals can take their minds off their pain and reduce their stress levels. In addition, engaging in creative activities can help improve dexterity, hand-eye coordination, and overall range of motion.

However, for those with arthritis, adapting their creative practice to their physical limitations is important. This may involve using different materials or tools, taking breaks as needed, and finding ways to work around any mobility issues.

For example, individuals with arthritis in their hands may need to use adaptive tools, such as ergonomic paintbrushes or pens with a larger grip. Those with arthritis in their hips or knees may need to find ways to work while seated or modify their movements to avoid discomfort.

Fortunately, there are many resources available for those looking to adapt their creative practice. Occupational therapists can provide guidance on using adaptive tools and techniques, and many online communities offer support and inspiration for those with arthritis.

It's also important to find inspiration and motivation in a way that works for each individual. For some, it may be joining a local art class or music group. For others, it may be starting a new project at home or finding inspiration in nature or the world around them.

It's important to remember that creativity is not just about creating something tangible. Engaging in creative activities can also involve immersing oneself in books, films, and other forms of art that provide inspiration and mental stimulation.

In addition to the physical and mental benefits, finding inspiration and motivation through creativity can also lead to a sense of accomplishment and pride in one's work. This can help boost self-esteem and provide a sense of purpose and meaning in life.

Of course, it's important to listen to one's body and take breaks as needed. Overexertion can lead to further pain and discomfort, so pacing oneself and taking frequent breaks is key.

Chapter Thirty-Two

Complementary and Integrative Medicine

Complementary and integrative medicine (CIM) refers to a group of diverse health care practices and products that are not part of mainstream medical care but are used alongside conventional medicine to support and enhance health and well-being. CIM can be especially beneficial for individuals with chronic conditions such as arthritis, as it can help manage symptoms and improve overall quality of life.

CIM encompasses a wide range of practices, including acupuncture, massage therapy, herbal medicine, dietary supplements, and mind-body therapies such as meditation and yoga. While some CIM therapies have been studied more extensively than others, many have shown promising results in reducing pain, inflammation, and other arthritis symptoms.

One CIM practice that has gained significant attention for its potential benefits in arthritis management is acupuncture. This traditional Chinese medicine technique involves inserting thin needles into specific points on the body to stimulate healing and alleviate pain. Acupuncture has been found to be effective in reducing pain and improving joint function in people with osteoarthritis and rheumatoid arthritis. It may also help reduce inflammation and improve blood flow to affected joints.

Another CIM practice that has shown promise in arthritis management is massage therapy. Massage can help reduce pain and stiffness, improve range of motion, and promote relaxation and better sleep. In particular, myofascial release massage, which involves applying gentle pressure to tight areas of muscle and connective tissue, may be especially beneficial for individuals with arthritis.

Herbal medicine is another form of CIM that has been used for centuries to treat various health conditions, including arthritis. Certain herbs and spices such as turmeric, ginger, and willow bark contain compounds that have anti-inflammatory properties and may help reduce pain and inflammation in individuals with arthritis. However, it is important to note that herbal remedies should be used with caution and under the guidance of a qualified health care provider, as they can interact with medications and may not be safe for everyone.

Dietary supplements, such as glucosamine and chondroitin, are also commonly used by individuals with arthritis to support joint health. While research on the effectiveness of these supplements is mixed, some studies have found that they may help reduce pain and stiffness in individuals with osteoarthritis. It is important to note, however, that not all supplements are created equal, and it is important to choose high-quality products and to speak with a healthcare provider before starting any new supplement regimen.

Mind-body therapies such as meditation and yoga have also been found to be helpful in managing arthritis symptoms. These practices can help reduce stress and promote relaxation, which can in turn help reduce pain and inflammation. Additionally, yoga can help improve joint flexibility and range of motion, which may be especially beneficial for individuals with arthritis.

The role of complementary therapies

Arthritis is a chronic condition that affects millions of people worldwide. While there are conventional medical treatments for arthritis, such as medication and surgery, some people turn to complementary and integrative medicine (CIM) as a way to manage their symptoms. CIM is a term that encompasses a range of therapies and practices that are not considered conventional medicine but are used alongside or in conjunction with conventional treatments.

The goal of CIM is to improve the overall well-being of a person by addressing the physical, emotional, and spiritual aspects of their health. There are several types of CIM therapies that may be helpful for arthritis, including acupuncture, massage therapy, chiropractic, yoga, and meditation.

Acupuncture is a traditional Chinese medicine practice that involves inserting thin needles into specific points on the body. Acupuncture is thought to help reduce inflammation and pain, which are common symptoms of arthritis. According to the National Center for Complementary and Integrative Health (NCCIH), several studies have found that acupuncture may be helpful for reducing pain and improving function in people with osteoarthritis, rheumatoid arthritis, and fibromyalgia.

Massage therapy involves manipulating the soft tissues of the body, such as muscles and tendons, with hands-on techniques. Massage therapy may help reduce pain and stiffness in people with arthritis by increasing blood flow to the affected area and promoting relaxation. According to the Arthritis Foundation, several studies have found that massage therapy may be helpful for reducing pain and improving function in people with arthritis.

Chiropractic care involves using hands-on techniques to manipulate the spine and other joints in the body. Chiropractic care may help reduce pain and stiffness in people with arthritis by improving joint mobility and alignment. According to the American Chiropractic Association, several studies have found that chiropractic care may be helpful for reducing pain and improving function in people with osteoarthritis.

Yoga is a mind-body practice that involves physical postures, breathing exercises, and meditation. Yoga may help reduce pain and improve function in people with arthritis by increasing flexibility, strength, and relaxation. According to the NCCIH, several studies have found that yoga may be helpful for reducing pain and improving function in people with osteoarthritis and rheumatoid arthritis.

Meditation is a practice that involves focusing the mind on a specific object, thought, or activity to achieve a state of relaxation and inner peace. Meditation may help reduce stress, which is a common trigger for arthritis symptoms. According to the Arthritis Foundation, several studies have found that meditation may be helpful for reducing pain and improving function in people with arthritis.

It's important to note that CIM therapies are not a replacement for conventional medical treatments for arthritis. However, they may be used alongside conventional treatments as a way to manage symptoms and improve overall well-being. It's also important to talk to a healthcare provider before starting any CIM therapy to ensure it's safe and appropriate for you.

In addition to the therapies mentioned above, there are several other CIM practices that may be helpful for arthritis, including:

1. Dietary supplements: Some dietary supplements, such as glucosamine and chondroitin, may help reduce pain and improve joint function in people with osteoarthritis.

2. Mind-body therapies: Mind-body therapies, such as biofeedback and hypnotherapy, may help reduce stress and pain in people with arthritis.

3. Herbal remedies: Some herbs, such as turmeric and ginger, may have anti-inflammatory properties that may help reduce pain and stiffness in people with arthritis.

While CIM therapies may be helpful for arthritis, it's important to approach them with caution. Some CIM therapies may not be backed by strong scientific evidence, and some may even be harmful if used improperly. It's also important to seek out qualified practitioners who are trained in the specific CIM therapy you're interested in.

Integrating conventional and alternative treatments

Arthritis is a common condition that affects millions of people worldwide, causing pain, stiffness, and swelling in the joints. While conventional treatments such as medication, physical therapy, and surgery can be effective in managing symptoms, some people may choose to explore alternative therapies to complement their treatment plan. This approach is known as integrative medicine, which combines conventional medicine with complementary and alternative therapies to promote overall health and well-being. Below we will discuss the benefits and challenges of integrating conventional and alternative treatments for arthritis.

Complementary and alternative therapies encompass a wide range of practices, including acupuncture, massage, chiropractic, herbal medicine, meditation, and yoga. These therapies are considered "complementary" because they are used alongside conventional treatments, and "alternative" because they may be used in place of conventional treatments. Many people with arthritis turn to these therapies because they offer a natural, holistic approach to managing pain and improving overall health.

One of the benefits of complementary and alternative therapies is that they can help manage pain and improve mobility without the use of medications that may have side effects. For example, acupuncture is a form of traditional Chinese medicine that involves inserting needles into specific points on the body to stimulate the flow of energy and promote healing. Studies have shown that acupuncture can be effective in reducing pain and improving joint function in people with osteoarthritis, rheumatoid arthritis, and fibromyalgia.

Massage therapy is another complementary therapy that can help manage pain and stiffness in the joints. Massage works by increasing circulation and reducing muscle tension, which can improve joint mobility and reduce pain. Chiropractic care, which involves the manipulation of the spine and joints, can also be effective in reducing pain and improving joint function.

Herbal medicine is another complementary therapy that is used to manage arthritis symptoms. Herbs such as turmeric, ginger, and boswellia have anti-inflammatory properties and can help reduce joint pain and swelling. However, it is important to note that herbal remedies can interact with medications and should be used with caution.

Meditation and yoga are mindfulness-based practices that can help manage stress and improve overall well-being. Stress can exacerbate arthritis symptoms, so learning how to manage stress through these practices can be beneficial. Yoga, in particular, can help improve joint mobility, balance, and strength.

While complementary and alternative therapies can be beneficial in managing arthritis symptoms, there are some challenges to integrating these therapies with conventional treatments. One challenge is that some complementary therapies are not covered by insurance, which can make them cost-prohibitive for some people. Additionally, some complementary therapies may not be suitable for everyone, and it is important to consult with a healthcare professional before starting any new therapy.

Another challenge is that some complementary therapies may interact with conventional treatments or have their own side effects. For example, some herbal remedies can interact with medications and may not be safe for people with certain health conditions. It is important to talk with a healthcare professional before starting any new therapy to ensure that it is safe and effective for you.

Finding a balance between approaches

Arthritis is a complex condition that affects millions of people worldwide. While conventional treatments like medication and physical therapy are often the first line of defense against arthritis symptoms, many people are turning to complementary and alternative therapies to manage their condition. These approaches can include anything from dietary supplements to acupuncture, and while they may not always be backed by extensive scientific research, many people find them to be effective.

One of the primary benefits of complementary and alternative therapies is that they can provide a more holistic approach to managing arthritis. While conventional treatments tend to focus on addressing the physical symptoms of the condition, complementary therapies can address a range of factors that can contribute to arthritis, including stress, anxiety, and emotional wellbeing.

One of the most popular complementary therapies for arthritis is massage therapy. Massage has been shown to be effective in reducing pain, stiffness, and muscle tension in people with arthritis. Massage can also help to increase range of motion, improve circulation, and promote relaxation. While massage is generally safe for most people with arthritis, it is important to find a qualified massage therapist who has experience working with people with the condition.

Another popular alternative therapy for arthritis is acupuncture. Acupuncture involves the insertion of thin needles into specific points on the body, and it has been used for centuries to treat a variety of health conditions. While the research on acupuncture for arthritis is somewhat mixed, many people find it to be effective in reducing pain and improving function. Like massage therapy, it is important to find a qualified acupuncturist who has experience working with people with arthritis.

Dietary supplements are also a popular complementary therapy for arthritis. While there is limited scientific evidence to support the use of supplements for arthritis, many people find that they can be effective in reducing inflammation and pain. Some of the most commonly used supplements for arthritis include omega-3 fatty acids, glucosamine and chondroitin, and turmeric. It is important to talk to your healthcare provider before starting any new supplements, as they can interact with other medications and may not be appropriate for everyone.

Mind-body practices like yoga and meditation are also gaining popularity as complementary therapies for arthritis. These practices have been shown to be effective in reducing stress and anxiety, which can exacerbate arthritis symptoms. Additionally, they can help to improve flexibility, strength, and balance, which can help to reduce the risk of falls and injury. Like with other complementary therapies, it is important to find an experienced instructor who can tailor the practice to your specific needs.

While complementary and alternative therapies can be effective in managing arthritis symptoms, it is important to remember that they should not be used as a substitute for conventional medical treatment. Rather, they can be used in conjunction with conventional treatments to provide a more holistic approach to managing the condition.

It is also important to approach complementary and alternative therapies with an open mind, but also a critical eye. While many of these approaches can be effective, not all of them are backed by solid scientific evidence. It is important to do your research and talk to your healthcare provider before starting any new therapies, as they can interact with other medications and may not be appropriate for everyone.

Ultimately, finding the right balance between conventional and complementary treatments for arthritis will depend on your individual needs and preferences. By exploring a range of approaches and working closely with your healthcare provider, you can find a treatment plan that works best for you and helps you to manage your arthritis symptoms effectively.

Chapter Thirty-Three

Arthritis Advocacy and Awareness

Arthritis is a debilitating condition that affects millions of people worldwide. It is a condition that causes inflammation and pain in the joints, making it difficult for sufferers to perform everyday tasks. Unfortunately, arthritis is often misunderstood, leading to stigma and a lack of awareness. This is why advocacy and awareness are crucial for individuals living with arthritis. Below we will explore the importance of arthritis advocacy and awareness, the impact it can have on the lives of those with the condition, and the ways in which individuals can get involved in advocating for arthritis.

Advocacy for arthritis involves raising awareness about the condition, improving access to treatment and care, and promoting policies and laws that benefit people with arthritis. One of the main goals of arthritis advocacy is to reduce the stigma associated with the condition. By raising awareness and understanding, people can begin to see arthritis as a legitimate condition and not just a sign of aging or weakness. Advocacy also aims to improve access to treatment and care, as many people with arthritis struggle to afford or access the medical care they need. This can include lobbying for better insurance coverage, increasing funding for research, and improving access to specialists.

Arthritis awareness is another crucial aspect of advocacy. By increasing public knowledge about arthritis, individuals can learn about the symptoms, causes, and treatment options available for the condition. This can lead to earlier diagnosis and treatment, which can prevent further joint damage and improve overall quality of life. Awareness can also help to reduce stigma, as people begin to understand the realities of living with arthritis and the challenges that come with the condition.

Advocacy and awareness efforts can have a significant impact on the lives of people living with arthritis. For instance, by advocating for more research and funding, individuals can help to develop new treatments and therapies for arthritis. This can lead to better pain management, improved quality of life, and even the possibility of a cure. Advocacy can also lead to policy changes that benefit people with arthritis, such as better access to healthcare or improved disability accommodations.

Individuals can get involved in arthritis advocacy and awareness efforts in several ways. One way is to participate in arthritis-related events, such as walks or fundraisers, which help to raise awareness and funds for research and treatment. Another way is to contact local and national representatives and advocate for policies and laws that benefit people with arthritis. Individuals can also join arthritis advocacy organizations, such as the Arthritis Foundation, which advocates for research, treatment, and policy changes that benefit people with arthritis.

In addition to advocacy and awareness, individuals with arthritis can also benefit from self-advocacy. This involves taking an active role in managing their own care and treatment, such as by working with doctors to develop treatment plans that meet their needs, or by seeking out information about arthritis and treatment options. Self-advocacy can also involve advocating for accommodations at work or in other settings to help manage the challenges of living with arthritis.

The importance of advocacy

Arthritis is a chronic condition that affects millions of people worldwide. It can cause pain, stiffness, and swelling in the joints, which can lead to reduced mobility and quality of life. Despite the prevalence of arthritis, there is still a lot of misinformation and stigma surrounding the condition. This is where arthritis advocacy and awareness come in. Advocacy is about speaking up and promoting change, while awareness is about educating people and raising public consciousness about an issue. Below we will explore the importance of arthritis advocacy and awareness.

One of the main reasons why arthritis advocacy is crucial is that it helps to ensure that people with arthritis have access to the resources and support they need to manage their condition. This includes access to healthcare services, medication, and assistive devices such as mobility aids and orthotics. Advocacy can also help to ensure that people with arthritis are not discriminated against in the workplace or denied access to education and other opportunities. By speaking up about their experiences, people with arthritis can raise awareness of the challenges they face and advocate for change.

Another important aspect of arthritis advocacy is the need to promote research into the causes, treatments, and prevention of arthritis. Despite the fact that arthritis is a common condition, there is still much that we do not know about it. By advocating for increased funding and support for research, we can gain a better understanding of the condition and develop more effective treatments.

Arthritis awareness is also essential because it helps to combat the stigma and misconceptions surrounding the condition. Many people believe that arthritis only affects older people or that it is a minor inconvenience rather than a serious health condition. However, arthritis can affect people of all ages and can have a significant impact on their lives. By raising awareness of the condition, we can help to dispel myths and educate people about the realities of living with arthritis.

Furthermore, arthritis awareness can help people to recognize the symptoms of the condition and seek appropriate treatment. Many people with arthritis delay seeking medical attention, either because they are unaware of the symptoms or because they are hesitant to seek help. By educating the public about the signs of arthritis and the importance of early diagnosis and treatment, we can help more people to access the care they need.

There are several ways in which individuals and organizations can get involved in arthritis advocacy and awareness. One of the most effective ways is to share personal stories and experiences. By speaking openly about their experiences with arthritis, people can help to raise awareness of the condition and the challenges it poses. Social media is also an excellent tool for advocacy and awareness-raising, allowing people to share information, connect with others, and promote events and initiatives.

Organizations such as arthritis foundations and patient advocacy groups play an important role in advocacy and awareness. These organizations work to promote research, improve access to care, and raise public consciousness about arthritis. They also provide support and resources to people with arthritis and their families, helping them to manage the condition and live full and active lives.

Becoming an arthritis ambassador

Arthritis is a debilitating condition that affects millions of people worldwide. It can cause severe pain, stiffness, and reduced mobility, making it challenging to perform everyday activities. Arthritis is not only physically taxing but also mentally and emotionally draining. Coping with arthritis can be overwhelming, and the support and guidance of an arthritis ambassador can be invaluable.

Becoming an arthritis ambassador is a great way to raise awareness and advocate for those living with arthritis. An arthritis ambassador is someone who takes an active role in promoting arthritis education and advocacy. They work to increase awareness of arthritis, advocate for research funding, and support others with arthritis.

The role of an arthritis ambassador is vital in ensuring that those with arthritis receive the care and support they need. By raising awareness of arthritis, ambassadors help others understand the condition's impact and the need for research and funding. They also work to promote access to effective treatments and support services for those living with arthritis.

To become an arthritis ambassador, there are several things that you can do. Firstly, educating yourself about arthritis is critical. By understanding the condition, you can help others recognize its impact and the importance of taking care of your joints. There are numerous resources available to learn about arthritis, including books, online courses, and local support groups.

Once you have an understanding of the condition, the next step is to raise awareness. This can be done through social media, hosting fundraising events, or by participating in local community events. You can also reach out to local health organizations and offer to speak about arthritis and the need for support and funding.

Advocacy is another essential component of being an arthritis ambassador. This involves reaching out to policymakers and urging them to support research and funding for arthritis. It also involves supporting legislation that benefits those with arthritis, such as insurance coverage for arthritis medications and therapies.

Finally, being a supportive presence for those living with arthritis is crucial. This can involve offering emotional support, helping them find effective treatments, and encouraging them to participate in support groups and community events.

Becoming an arthritis ambassador is a rewarding experience that can make a significant difference in the lives of those living with arthritis. By raising awareness, advocating for research and funding, and supporting others, ambassadors help improve the lives of those affected by arthritis.

Supporting arthritis research and awareness efforts

Arthritis is a condition that affects millions of people worldwide, and yet it is often misunderstood and underrepresented in research and public awareness campaigns. As such, it is important for individuals to become advocates for arthritis research and awareness efforts, in order to improve the lives of those living with arthritis and promote progress in the field.

There are a number of ways to support arthritis research and awareness efforts. One of the most important is to become informed about the condition and its impact on people's lives. This means staying up-to-date with the latest research, reading about the experiences of others with arthritis, and educating oneself about the resources available for managing the condition.

Another important way to support arthritis research and awareness is to become involved in advocacy efforts. This can involve contacting legislators and policymakers to advocate for increased funding for arthritis research, joining advocacy organizations and participating in their efforts to promote awareness and support for people with arthritis, and participating in events and campaigns designed to raise awareness about the condition.

There are also many opportunities to contribute to arthritis research efforts directly. For example, individuals can participate in clinical trials or studies to help researchers better understand the condition and develop new treatments. They can also donate to organizations and research institutions working on arthritis research, or even start their own fundraising efforts to support the cause.

In addition to these more formal methods of supporting arthritis research and awareness, there are many ways to promote awareness and understanding of the condition in everyday life. For example, individuals can share their own experiences with arthritis with others, raise awareness through social media or other online platforms, and participate in community events and activities that promote arthritis awareness and support.

Ultimately, the key to supporting arthritis research and awareness efforts is to remain informed, engaged, and active in promoting progress in the field. By working together, individuals can help to improve the lives of those living with arthritis and pave the way for a better future for all those affected by this condition.

Chapter Thirty-Four

Setting and Achieving Goals

Arthritis is a chronic disease that affects the joints, causing pain, stiffness, and swelling. It can be a challenging condition to manage, but with proper self-care and goal-setting, it's possible to maintain a good quality of life. Setting and achieving goals is an essential aspect of managing arthritis. It can help to improve overall health, maintain independence, and provide a sense of purpose and accomplishment.

Here are some tips for setting and achieving goals with arthritis:

Start Small

When setting goals, it's important to start small. Set achievable goals that are realistic and within reach. Setting big goals can be overwhelming, and if they're not achieved, it can be discouraging. Breaking down larger goals into smaller, more manageable steps can make them feel more achievable.

For example, if your goal is to walk for 30 minutes every day, start by walking for five or ten minutes a day and gradually increase the duration over time. This approach will help you build confidence and motivation as you see progress toward your goal.

Be Specific

Setting specific goals is important because it helps to define what you want to achieve. Specific goals help to focus your efforts and give you direction.

Instead of setting a vague goal like "I want to exercise more," set a specific goal like "I want to walk for 30 minutes three times a week."

Being specific helps you to measure progress and adjust your efforts accordingly. It also helps to keep you accountable and motivated.

Set Realistic Timelines

Setting a deadline for your goals can help to keep you motivated and focused. However, it's important to set realistic timelines. Achieving goals takes time, and setting unrealistic deadlines can lead to frustration and discouragement.

It's also important to be flexible with your timelines. Arthritis can be unpredictable, and some days may be better than others. If you need to adjust your timeline, be kind to yourself and make the necessary changes.

Be Flexible

Flexibility is key when managing arthritis. You may need to adjust your goals or approach based on how you're feeling. It's important to be flexible and make changes as needed.

For example, if your goal is to attend a yoga class twice a week, but you're having a flare-up, you may need to adjust your schedule or try a different type of exercise. Being flexible and open to new approaches can help you to achieve your goals in a way that's best for you.

Celebrate Small Wins

Achieving goals takes time, and it's important to celebrate small wins along the way. Celebrating small wins can help to keep you motivated and focused on your overall goal.

For example, if your goal is to walk for 30 minutes every day, celebrate when you're able to walk for five minutes without pain. Celebrating small wins helps to build confidence and momentum toward your larger goal.

Get Support

Managing arthritis can be challenging, and it's important to have a support system in place. Getting support from family, friends, or a healthcare professional can help to keep you motivated and accountable.

For example, if your goal is to eat a healthy diet, enlist the help of a friend or family member to meal prep with you. Having someone to share your journey with can make the process more enjoyable and less daunting.

In addition, talking to a healthcare professional can help to ensure that your goals are safe and appropriate for your condition. They can also provide guidance and support as you work toward your goals.

Goal-setting for arthritis management

Arthritis is a chronic condition that affects millions of people worldwide. It can be a painful and disabling condition, and it can significantly impact a person's quality of life. However, there are ways to manage the symptoms of arthritis and improve overall well-being. One of the most effective ways to do this is by setting and achieving goals.

Goal-setting is an essential aspect of arthritis management. Goals can provide a sense of purpose and motivation, and they can help individuals take control of their condition. When it comes to managing arthritis, goals should be specific, measurable, attainable, relevant, and time-bound (SMART). This means that they should be clear, measurable, achievable, relevant to the person's situation, and have a deadline for completion.

There are different types of goals that people with arthritis can set. These include:

1. Pain management goals: These goals are focused on reducing pain and discomfort. Examples of pain management goals include practicing relaxation techniques, taking medications as prescribed, and incorporating physical therapy into the daily routine.

2. Mobility goals: These goals are focused on improving movement and flexibility. Examples of mobility goals include increasing range of motion in affected joints, participating in low-impact exercise, and using assistive devices such as braces or canes.

3. Lifestyle goals: These goals are focused on making lifestyle changes that can improve overall health and well-being. Examples of lifestyle goals include eating a healthy diet, getting regular exercise, quitting smoking, and reducing stress.

4. Social goals: These goals are focused on maintaining social connections and participating in activities that bring joy and fulfillment. Examples of social goals include joining a support group, volunteering, and pursuing hobbies or interests.

When setting goals, it is important to consider the individual's specific needs and limitations. For example, a person with severe arthritis may not be able to participate in high-impact exercise, so low-impact options such as swimming or yoga may be more appropriate. Additionally, goals should be flexible and adjustable as needed. If a person experiences a setback or change in condition, their goals may need to be adjusted to reflect the new situation.

To achieve arthritis management goals, there are several strategies that can be helpful. These include:

5. Breaking down goals into smaller steps: Large goals can be overwhelming, so breaking them down into smaller, manageable steps can make them more achievable.

6. Tracking progress: Keeping track of progress can be motivating and help individuals stay on track towards their goals. This can be done through journaling, using an app, or working with a healthcare provider to monitor progress.

7. Celebrating successes: Celebrating successes, no matter how small, can help individuals stay motivated and maintain a positive outlook.

8. Seeking support: Having a support system can be invaluable when working towards goals. This can include family and friends, healthcare providers, and support groups.

9. Staying positive: Maintaining a positive attitude can help individuals overcome obstacles and stay motivated towards achieving their goals.

Overcoming setbacks and obstacles

Arthritis is a chronic condition that can be accompanied by pain, stiffness, and decreased mobility. The symptoms of arthritis can be unpredictable and can vary from day to day. This unpredictability can make it difficult to maintain a consistent routine and achieve goals. However, there are strategies that can help individuals with arthritis overcome setbacks and obstacles to achieve their goals.

One of the first steps in overcoming setbacks and obstacles is to acknowledge that they will happen. Arthritis symptoms can flare up unexpectedly, and it is important to be prepared for these setbacks. It can be helpful to have a backup plan in place for when symptoms interfere with goal-oriented activities. This may mean having a contingency plan for exercise routines or a backup plan for important events that cannot be missed.

Another key strategy for overcoming setbacks and obstacles is to be adaptable. Arthritis symptoms can vary greatly from day to day, and it is important to be flexible in adapting to these changes. This may mean adjusting goals or expectations based on symptoms or finding alternative ways to achieve a goal.

Stress management is another important tool for overcoming setbacks and obstacles. Stress can exacerbate arthritis symptoms, and it is important to manage stress levels in order to maintain good overall health. Techniques such as deep breathing, meditation, and yoga can be helpful in managing stress levels and reducing the impact of stress on arthritis symptoms.

It can also be helpful to seek support from others when facing setbacks and obstacles. Arthritis support groups can be a valuable source of support and encouragement. Friends and family can also provide emotional support and assistance with tasks when arthritis symptoms are particularly challenging.

In addition, it is important to maintain a positive attitude when faced with setbacks and obstacles. A positive outlook can help individuals with arthritis maintain motivation and focus on achieving their goals. Celebrating small successes along the way can also be a helpful strategy in maintaining a positive attitude and staying motivated.

Finally, it can be helpful to work with a healthcare professional or arthritis specialist to develop a plan for managing symptoms and achieving goals. This may involve medication management, physical therapy, or other treatments. A healthcare professional can also provide guidance on safe and effective exercise and activity modifications that can help individuals with arthritis achieve their goals while minimizing the risk of injury.

Celebrating achievements and milestones

Arthritis can be a challenging condition that affects a person's ability to perform daily activities and achieve their goals. However, it is important to celebrate achievements and milestones in the face of such challenges. Doing so can boost self-esteem, provide motivation, and improve overall well-being.

Achievements and milestones can be big or small, and they are unique to each person. For someone with arthritis, simply being able to walk to the end of the block without pain can be a significant accomplishment. Others may celebrate milestones like completing a 5K run, finishing a home improvement project, or achieving a career goal. Whatever the achievement or milestone may be, it is important to recognize and celebrate it.

Celebrating achievements and milestones can have numerous benefits for people with arthritis. Firstly, it can boost self-esteem and confidence. When people achieve something they have been working towards, it can provide a sense of accomplishment and pride. This can help to improve self-esteem and give people the confidence to tackle new challenges.

Celebrating achievements and milestones can also provide motivation. When people see the progress they have made, it can inspire them to continue working towards their goals. It can also help to reinforce the importance of self-care and following a treatment plan.

Furthermore, celebrating achievements and milestones can improve overall well-being. It can provide a sense of happiness and satisfaction, which can help to combat feelings of depression and anxiety that can often be associated with chronic conditions like arthritis. It can also foster a sense of community and support, as loved ones can celebrate these achievements with the person with arthritis.

While celebrating achievements and milestones is important, it is also important to acknowledge the setbacks and obstacles that may arise. Living with arthritis can be unpredictable, and setbacks can occur despite a person's best efforts. When these setbacks happen, it is important to recognize and address them, rather than ignoring or dismissing them.

Overcoming setbacks and obstacles can be challenging, but it is important to remember that they are a normal part of the journey. It may be helpful to seek support from loved ones, healthcare providers, or support groups. It is also important to practice self-care and prioritize activities that help manage arthritis symptoms, like exercise, healthy eating, and stress management techniques.

In addition to celebrating achievements and milestones, it can also be helpful to set new goals. This can provide a sense of purpose and direction, and can help to keep people motivated and engaged in their treatment plan. When setting goals, it is important to be realistic and specific. Goals that are too vague or unrealistic can lead to frustration and disappointment.

When working towards new goals, it is also important to track progress and make adjustments as needed. This can help people stay on track and make meaningful progress towards their goals. It can also help to break larger goals down into smaller, more manageable steps.

SD - #0028 - 140926 - C0 - 229/152/15 - PB - 9781776967940 - Matt Lamination